T·H·E
CANDIDA
CONTROL
COOKBOOK

GAIL BURTON

With an Introduction by
MICHAEL E. ROSENBAUM, M.D.

Foreword by
Gail Nielsen
Founding Director of the Candida
Research and Information Foundation

Third Edition
(Contains many Revisions and Updates . . . Recipes, Addresses)

Aslan Publishing
Fairfield, Connecticut

Published by
Aslan Publishing
2490 Black Rock Turnpike, #342
Faifield, CT 06432
USA
203-372-0300

For a free catalog of all our titles, or to order more copies
of this book please call 1-800-786-5427

Aslan Publishing—Our Mission

Aslan Publishing offers readers a window to the soul via well-crafted and practical self-help books, inspirational books and modern day parables. Our mission is to publish books that uplift one's mind, body and spirit.

Living one's spirituality in business, relationships, and personal growth is the underlying purpose of our publishing company, and the meaning behind our name Aslan Publishing. We see the word "Aslan" as a metaphor for living spiritually in a physical world.

Aslan means "lion" in several Middle Eastern languages. The most famous "Aslan" is a lion in *The Chronicles of Narnia* by C. S. Lewis. In these stories, Aslan is the Messiah, the One who appears at critical points in the story in order to point human beings in the right direction. Aslan doesn't preach, he acts. His actions are an inherent expression of who he is.

We hope to point the way toward joyful, satisfying and healthy relationships with oneself and with others. Our purpose is to make a real difference in the everyday lives of our readers.

Barbara H. Levine   Harold Levine

Library of Congress Cataloging-in-Publication Data

Burton, Gail.
    The candida control cookbook : what you should know and what you should eat to manage yeast infections / Gail Burton ; with an introduction by Michael E. Rosenbaum ; foreword by Gail Nielsen. — Rev. ed.
        p. cm.
    Includes bibliographical references and index.
    ISBN 0-944031-67-6
    1. Candidiasis—Diet therapy—Recipes. 2. Candidiasis—Prevention. 3. Yeast-free diet—Recipes. I. Title.
    RC123.C3B87 1993
    616.9'69—dc20   92-33404
                                                                  CIP

Third Edition
Third Printing, 2000
Updated Appendix
Printed in USA

ACKNOWLEDGEMENTS

I wish to thank the following people who helped to make this book a reality instead of a dream:

Michael E. Rosenbaum, M.D., specializing in allergies, nutrition and preventive medicine, co-author of *Super Supplements,* and *Solving the Puzzle of Chronic Fatigue Syndrome*, for his tremendous support, and technical and content advice.

Gail Nielsen, Founding Director of the Candida Research and Information Foundation, for her generous time, information and content advice.

Millie Levin, artist, for her clever illustrations.

Ida W. Klinger, M.S.W., for her undying faith in me, and for her recipes, test-baking and cooking.

My dear family and friends, too numerous to mention, who supported me with their love and recipe testing.

The many *Candida* sufferers who made me realize the necessity of this book.

To

Michael E. Rosenbaum, M.D.

*With his knowledge and help,
I am able to live again.*

Contents

Foreword

So much of what is pleasurable in our lives revolves around food. Yet this very social function of eating can become a nightmare, a thing that dominates the very existence not only of the *Candida* patient, but also of most of the chronically ill. As a *Candida* patient herself, Gail Burton, a gourmet cook and writer of a gourmet foods column in a local newspaper, put her skills to work to take the drudgery out of cooking and eating for the *Candida* patient, specifically, and the chronically ill, in general, with this delightful cookbook.

It was established as early as 1923 by J. A. Buchanan, M.D., that a particular diet was essential for the recovery of the *Candida* patient ("Significance of Yeast in Stomach and Intestines," *International Journal of Medical Surgery* 43 [1930]: 14–17). In recent years, since the work of C. Orian Truss, M.D., revealed the *Candida* organism as a major cause of chronic unwellness, the patients themselves have noted that a low-carbohydrate diet is crucial in attaining and maintaining health. The greatest complaint from patients has been that the diet is the single most important and yet the most difficult part of treatment.

The Candida *Control Cookbook* was designed to put joy back into our daily lives through cooking and eating. Bon appétit!

—GAIL NIELSEN, M.S.,
Founding Director,
Candida Research and
Information Foundation

Note: For details on the Candida Research and Information Foundation, see Appendix C.

xi

Preface

I want you to know from firsthand experience that sensitivity to *Candida*, an internal yeast, need not keep you from enjoying meals, entertaining, and life!

After suffering ill health for over ten years, it was my good fortune to find Dr. Michael Rosenbaum, of Corte Madera, California, who specializes in preventive medicine, allergies, and nutrition. He suspected and correctly diagnosed my condition as *Candida*. It is essential to have the yeast condition diagnosed and supervised by a health care professional.

Along with a medically controlled treatment program, Dr. Rosenbaum gave me a special diet to follow. However, it was difficult for me to adhere to because it seemed so strict. Yet, when I deviated from the diet, my symptoms recurred. I soon realized that in order to achieve good results, I had to stick to the diet. And to accomplish this, I needed to have good recipes!

After much research and experimentation, I created recipes not only for myself and my family but for entertaining as well. I learned from the Candida Research and Information Foundation that there are millions of *Candida* or yeast-sensitive people all over the world and that a good cookbook for yeast control was greatly needed.

The Candida *Control Cookbook* will whet your appetite with over 150 delicious recipes that use only ingredients permitted on the anti-*Candida* diet. I've provided introductory material, including lists of permitted and prohibited foods, a guide to the carbohydrate content of many foods, and a 14-day menu plan.

I've also provided lists of important dietary supplements and sources for some of the special ingredients you'll need; this information can be found in the appendixes.

Candida interferes with the body's immune responses and often results in sensitivity to many chemical formulas. Therefore, before you begin to use the recipes, consider having allergy tests administered by a health care professional. Beware, however: If you have extreme hypersensitivity, regular allergy testing may cause adverse reactions, so consult your health care professional or contact the Candida Research and Information Foundation for information (see Appendix C).

This cookbook advocates a low-carbohydrate diet. However, a health care professional should determine the amount of carbohydrate necessary for your particular condition.

If you *think in terms of foods you can have* as opposed to those you can't, *make good substitutions* for problem foods, and *are creative* with permitted foods, you should do well. *The* Candida *Control Diet Cookbook* has all the ingredients to make every meal a delight! Enjoy good health!

—GAIL BURTON
1989

Introduction

*T*here is mounting evidence that *Candida albicans*—the common yeast cell that is part of our body's normal flora—is not always an innocuous organism. Following decades of laboratory and clinical research about *Candida*, Dr. Orian Truss has alerted us to the prevalence of *Candida*-induced ailments.

Dr. Truss is convinced that there is an overgrowth of *Candida* in the population of affluent countries. This problem is attributed to the widespread use of broad-spectrum antibiotics, steroids, and birth control pills and a gross overconsumption of sweets.

Candida albicans has an unusual ability to survive on the warm, moist mucous membranes of the human body—predominantly in the digestive and genitourinary regions. It survives by adhering tenaciously to the cell membrane and by sending out cell projections, which penetrate the cell lining. Furthermore, *Candida* may release toxins that suppress the normal immune response that our bodies use to contain its growth. Theoretically, these toxins enter the bloodstream and contribute to numerous complaints: fatigue, aches and pains, emotional distress, impaired concentration, skin rashes, and digestive and genitourinary problems. This complex of symptoms has been called the *Candida* Toxicity Syndrome.

Treatment includes the use of antifungal medication in conjunction with a *Candida*-inhibition diet low in carbohydrates and fermented foods. Sufferers must stick to this diet for months and sometimes years because *Candida* is so difficult to eradicate.

Many patients complain that the diet is too stringent, boring, and tasteless. Enter Gail Burton!

Gail suffered from a long-standing digestive disorder that was resistant to conventional treatments. She obtained relief from the *Candida* treatment program.

An outstanding cook, Gail has devoted two years to devising and compiling gourmet *Candida*-inhibiting recipes that richly please the palate! To my delight, I have sampled and enjoyed several of these meals. I invite *you* to take delight in *The Candida Control Cookbook*.

—MICHAEL E. ROSENBAUM, M.D.
Corte Madera, California

Vital Information on *Candida*

What Is *Candida*?

Candida is a yeast infection. *Candida,* or Candidiasis, gets its name from *Candida albicans*, which are yeast that live in our mucous membranes. These yeast are harmless until certain factors cause them to become active and harmful, causing symptoms from head to toe.

What Factors Cause *Candida*?

Antibiotics, steroids, hormones, birth control pills, and even specific tranquilizers can cause *Candida*. These modern-day wonder drugs not only kill the bad bacteria, but the good as well. When the body doesn't have its good bacteria, there is no ammunition to fight disease. The immune system then becomes useless and vulnerable to worse infection and problems.

Stress is also a factor. If there is excessive or continued stress, it lowers the immune system and creates the perfect environment for *Candida*.

Too much sugar in the diet is also a factor because *Candida albicans* thrive on sugars and sweeteners. For further diet information, see the section in this book, "The Importance of the *Candida* Control Diet."

What Are the Symptoms of *Candida?*

The following symptoms could occur: extreme fatigue, gas or bloating after eating, poor digestion, recurring ear, nose, throat and respiratory infections, skin rashes, muscle and joint pains, insomnia, recurring headaches, dizziness, depression, anxiety, poor memory and concentration, recurring urinary and vaginal infections, thyroid dysfunction, irritable bowel syndrome, spastic colon, and allergies to foods, chemicals and mold. The list goes on and on.

The symptoms are so vast and diverse that many physicians may easily misdiagnose *Candida* and think that the patient is a hypochondriac or that emotional problems are causing the symptoms.

What Is the Magnitude of *Candida?*

At least one out of three people in the Western world have *Candida.* The disease affects not only women, but men, teenagers, children and babies. Women and men can get *Candida* from the above-mentioned factors and pass it on through sexual relations. Teenagers can become infected by *Candida* when they are routinely treated with antibiotics for acne. Children can get *Candida* from being treated with antibiotics for recurring ear and throat infections. Babies often get thrush—another form of *Candida*—from the infected mother.

Some people have mild forms of yeast infection while others have chronic conditions. There are *Candida* sufferers who are so ill that they can hardly work. Others cannot work at all and some are barely able to function.

Candida is connected to many diseases: multiple sclerosis, rheumatoid arthritis, Crohn's disease, lupus, Epstein-Barr, etc. Most cancer and AIDS patients have *Candida.*

What Is the Treatment Program for *Candida*?

Antifungals are important in treating *Candida*. There are many herbal remedies on the market to combat the infection. Some are mentioned in this book in Appendix A: "Nutritional Supplements for the Yeast Condition." There are also a few medications that treat *Candida*. Diflucan, a fairly new drug, has been found to be helpful in getting rid of *Candida*. However, it is important that a person be tested for adverse reactions and to be under the supervision of a health care professional while taking any medication.

It has also been found that acidophilus is helpful in building up the immune system. In addition, Vitamin C has been found to be beneficial by some *Candida* sufferers.

The most important part of the treatment program is the *Candida* Control Diet. The diet is designed to discourage yeast from thriving. The section, "The Importance of the *Candida* Control Diet: Problem Foods and Permitted Foods," explains in detail what foods should be avoided and what foods are allowed.

What Can Be Done to Prevent *Candida*?

Many times it is necessary to take an antibiotic for infection or steroids for inflammation. However, during treatment and possibly for a month or two afterward, it has been found that acidophilus as well as an antifungal are helpful in preventing *Candida*. Further information on these supplements is found in Appendix A.

The Importance of the *Candida* Control Diet

Your doctor may have diagnosed your symptoms as *Candida*, an internal yeast infection. Along with medication prescribed to destroy the yeast, he should also have suggested a yeast-control diet. This diet is necessary because certain foods promote yeast growth and undo the good any medication does. Therefore, for the treatment program to be successful, you should follow this special diet consistently. Because the diet may seem unduly strict, you should know the reasons; that way, you're less likely to become discouraged and decide to ignore it.

■ **No sugars or sweeteners** are allowed, because yeast thrive on them. **Avoid sweeteners such as dextrose, fructose, maltose, glucose, sorbital, aspartame, and NutraSweet.** Also **avoid any kind of malt, yeast, monosodium glutamate, citric acid, and any other additives** found in most canned and packaged dry and frozen foods; condiments and salad dressings; sauces; and vegetable, chicken, and beef bouillon seasonings. Become an expert label reader!

■ You will find no fruit recipes in this book other than ones using unsweetened cranberry concentrate. *Candida* sufferers should **avoid fruits** which are full of natural sugar, especially in the beginning stages of the treatment program. **Avoid any dried fruits** too because of mold, which collects during drying. In addition, **avoid any frozen or canned fruit or juices;** they contain yeast as well as natural sugar. Sadly, experience shows that most people who have recovered or improved, get symptoms again when fruit or juice is reintroduced into their diet.

■ **Wheat, barley and oat flours, bread and baked goods are prohibited** due to their high carbohydrate content as well as gluten, upon which Candida albicans thrive. In addition, baker's yeast should be avoided because many Candida sufferers are sensitive to it. However, yeast-free sourdough bread is beneficial because it contains strains of lactobacillus, an organism important for the proper digestion and absorption of complex carbohydrates and valuable nutrients.

■ **No dairy products, other than butter and eggs**, are allowed in the diet, because of their milk sugar, which feeds the yeast.

■ **Cheese** is omitted from the diet because it is made from mold-fermentation methods and may contain too many additives.

■ **All alcoholic beverages, especially wine and beer**, should be omitted during the treatment program, since wine is fermented with yeast and beer is brewed with a great deal of it. Other fermented items to avoid on the program include the following: **vinegar or any products made with vinegar, such as mustard, mayonnaise, pickles, and sauerkraut; soy sauce, tamari, and rice vinegar.** These items may cause problems due to their yeast content.

■ **Mushrooms** are not advised on the diet because they are fungi. Some patients are able to tolerate them, but it is best to wait until you are feeling up to experimenting before trying them.

■ **Common table salt** contains dextrose and many chemical additives. Therefore, use sea salt that is free of those ingredients.

■ **Black pepper** is hard to digest and is not recommended in cooking or seasoning of foods on the treatment program. However, **cayenne pepper** seems to promote digestion.

■ **Caffeine** is not permitted on the diet. In addition, **caffeinated and decaffeinated coffee, tea, and chocolate** are prohibited because of the mold that collects on the beans and leaves in the drying process. However, one cup a day of herbal tea is permitted. *Taheebo, Ipe Roxo, and Pau D'Arco teas (also known as La Pacho or Brazilian Herbal Tea)* are allowed, if you tolerate them, and are beneficial in combating yeast. La Pacho comes from the bark of trees grown free of fungi in the South American rain forests.

■ **Dried herbs** are not allowed on the diet due to the mold that collects on the leaves while drying, but fresh herbs are permitted. Garlic, in any form, is beneficial in combating yeast. Cloves also kill yeast.

■ Since fermentation may aggravate your symptoms, **cream of tartar** (made from the residue in wine barrels) should be avoided.

■ **Red meat** in general is hard to digest and recent research indicates that antibiotic-resistant strains of microorganisms can be spread by eating meats raised on steroids and antibiotics—basically, most commercially available meats. Therefore meat should be avoided in the early stages of treatment, unless it comes from animals that are raised without the use of growth hormones and antibiotics. Natural meats are available in some food stores at higher prices than those for meat that is processed in the standard way. If you cannot afford natural red meat, try chicken or fish. Some chickens are raised without chemicals or hormones; it is best to check with the producer. **Smoked or processed meats should also be avoided.**

■ Organically raised, fresh vegetables are preferable to other types of vegetables on your diet. They are available in most natural food stores.

■ **Melons and skins of fruit and vegetables** accumulate mold during growth. The Fusarium fungus grows on grapes and tomatoes. Scrub the skins of any vegetable or fruit, before peeling or cutting, to avoid ingesting mold.

■ **Peanuts and pistachios** are not permitted on the diet, since each harbors a particular type of fungus or parasite. Because of *aflatoxin*, the peanut fungus, **peanut oil** is not recommended for those on the treatment program.

The diet is low in carbohydrates initially. In general, *Candida* sufferers should keep their carbohydrate intake between **60 and 100 grams daily** during the early stages of treatment in order to inhibit yeast growth. However, again it must be emphasized that a health care professional should determine an individual's particular carbohydrate count.

The *Candida* Control Diet is shown in detail in the next section. The diet may not be a short-term affair. It may take a few months, several months, or much longer to regain your good health. However, many of your symptoms should disappear if, along with using medication to kill the yeast, you adhere to the diet with consistency. Good luck, good health, and good dining!

PROBLEM AND PERMITTED FOODS

PROBLEM FOODS	*PERMITTED FOODS*
Alcohol/other beverages:	
Beer, liquor, liqueur, wine, cider, malted milk, root beer, soda (any fermented, malted item or anything made with brewer's yeast)	Perrier, Calistoga water, soda water, seltzer, lime juice, lemon juice, Lemon Cooler, Mock Margaritas, or Perrier Cocktail (see index)
Breads and baked goods:	
All wheat and rye, baked and packaged products, breads, rolls, muffins, wheat tortillas, crackers (anything with baker's yeast, gluten or wheat)	Brown rice bread, Kamut, Millet, Rye, Spelt bread, bagels and pizza crust (all 100% wheat and yeast-free), sourdough bread (yeast-free)
Cereals:	
Oatmeal, all dry and hot cereals that contain malt and sweeteners	Oat and rice bran, Rice and Shine, puffed rice, millet and Quinoa

PROBLEM FOODS	PERMITTED FOODS
Cheeses:	
All hard cheese made from mold; all processed cheese, cream cheese, cottage cheese, ricotta	Raw cottage cheese (only if no digestive dysfunction)
Cornstarch:	
(for those sensitive to corn)	Arrowroot powder
Dairy products:	
Milk, buttermilk, whipped cream, sour cream, ice cream, toppings	Soy milk, nut milk, or egg whites (see "Dairy Substitutes"), fresh and not stored tofu (if tolerated), yogurt (if tolerated), eggs
Flavorings:	
All flavorings made with alcohol, sugar, and salt	Flavorings without alcohol, sugar, or salt
Flours:	
All barley, rye, and wheat flours (anything with gluten)	Amaranth flour, buckwheat flour, corn flour, garbanzo flour, millet flour, potato flour, rice flour, soy flour (all wheatless and without gluten)
Fruits:	
All fresh fruits, juices and melons (especially during first stages of treatment); all canned and dried fruits	Orange and lemon peels, if scrubbed well before cutting, peeling, or grating
Gelatins:	
All, including unflavored	Agar-agar (seaweed gelatin)

PROBLEM FOODS	PERMITTED FOODS
Herbs:	
All dried herbs, salt, pepper, Ac'cent, spices with yeast, sugar, sweeteners, monosodium glutamate (MSG), other chemicals (read labels carefully!)	Fresh herbs preferable, sea salt, garlic in any form, cloves, cayenne pepper
Margarines:	
All margarines, imitation spreads, and shortenings	*Heating or cooking:* 100% pure cold-pressed olive oil or Easy Clarified Butter (page 37) *Cold recipes or salads:* 100% pure cold-pressed olive oil, safflower oil (cold-pressed), sesame oil *Others:* Nut butters (see index)
Meats:	
Red meats, all processed and smoked meats, fish, and poultry	Natural red meats, poultry, and fish
Mushrooms:	
Because mushrooms are fungi, they may be a problem for some people. It may be best to avoid them until the condition improves.	
Noodles:	
All noodles containing wheat (gluten)	Bifun noodles (Chinese noodles, 100% wheat-free), corn noodles, Kuzu-Kiri (Japanese clear noodles), soba (Japanese noodles, 100% pure buckwheat)

PROBLEM FOODS	PERMITTED FOODS
Nuts and seeds:	
If the digestive system is sensitive, all nuts and seeds should be avoided; however, ground nuts are easier to digest than chopped, sliced, or slivered.	All nuts and seeds (in moderation)
Potatoes:	
Potato skins should be avoided	White, red, and sweet potatoes, yams (in moderation; all skins should be scrubbed well before peeling or slicing)
Rice and other grains:	
Barley, bulgur, oats, kosi (fermented rice), white rice	Brown rice, buckwheat, millet, quinoa, wild rice (in moderation)
Sugars and sweeteners:	
All sugars and sweeteners, corn and maple syrups, honey, molasses (read labels!)	100% Pure Vegetable Glycerine
Teas and coffees:	
All caffeinated and decaffeinated coffees and teas	Taheebo, Ipe Roxo, Pau d'Arco, and La Pacho teas (beneficial for treatment if tolerated), herb teas (in moderation)
Tomatoes:	
All canned tomatoes, tomato pastes, and sauces containing citric acid and/or sweeteners (read labels!)	Scrubbed and peeled fresh tomatoes, packaged tomatoes, tomato pastes and sauces without citric acid and/or sweeteners

PROBLEM FOODS	PERMITTED FOODS
Vegetables:	
Alfalfa sprouts, unpeeled and cooked beets and carrots	Peeled raw carrots, beans, beets, peas, and squash (all in moderation); all other vegetables (organic, fresh preferable), unlimited
Vinegar:	
All items made with vinegar (mayonnaise, mustard, salad dressings, sauces, marinated and pickled items), soy sauce, tamari (anything fermented)	Fresh lemon juice, Delicious Homemade Mayonnaise (page 145), salad dressings, sauces and marinades (all without vinegar)

The 14-Day
Candida Control
Menu Plan

*T*he purpose of this menu planner is to help you keep carbo-hydrate consumption between 60 and 100 grams daily in the beginning stages of treatment. As your condition improves, your carbohydrate consumption may be increased gradually. However, it is best to have a health care professional monitor your progress. Specific recipes follow. Substitute products and sources can be found in Appendix B. Snacks may be taken either in the middle of the afternoon or in the evening.

DAY 1

	Carbohydrate Grams
BREAKFAST	
⅓ cup dry oat bran, cooked	17
with ¼ cup Almond Milk	2
1 cup Taheebo Tea (optional)	0
LUNCH	
Shrimp-Stuffed Avocado	10
1 rice cake	8
Spring or mineral water	0

DAY 1 *(continued)*

DINNER

Chicken–Egg Drop Soup with Lemon	4
Cornish Hens à l'Orange	7
Wild Rice and Almonds	25
½ cup fresh scrubbed and cooked green beans	3

SNACK

5 brown rice crackers	7
1 cup Taheebo Tea (optional)	0
TOTAL CARBOHYDRATES	83

DAY 2

	Carbohydrate Grams
BREAKFAST	
1 Oat and Orange Muffin	15
1 cup herbal tea	0
LUNCH	
Curried Turkey and Almond Salad	5
1 rice cake	8
Spring or mineral water	0
DINNER	
Orange Roughy with Special Butter Sauce	3
Special Lemon Rice	22
Broccoli and Easy Hollandaise Sauce	5
2 cups scrubbed and chopped lettuce	4
2 tablespoons Creamy Herb Dressing	2
SNACK	
½ cup plain low-fat yogurt, sweetened with	12
100% Pure Vegetable Glycerine	0
TOTAL CARBOHYDRATES	76

DAY 3

	Carbohydrate Grams
BREAKFAST	
Eggplant Frittata	8
1 cup herbal tea	0
LUNCH	
Spinach and Egg Salad	7
2 tablespoons Creamy Herb Dressing	2
3 ounces tuna fish (packed in spring water)	0
1 rice cake	8
Iced chamomile	0
DINNER	
Baked Lemon Turkey Breast	7
Sweet Yam Casserole	14
1 cup scrubbed and shredded romaine lettuce	2
2 tablespoons Sweet Hot or Cold Tarragon Dressing	2
Royal Vanilla Custard	17
SNACK	
1 rice cake	8
1 cup Taheebo Tea (optional)	0
TOTAL CARBOHYDRATES	76

DAY 4

	Carbohydrate Grams
BREAKFAST	
1 heaping cup (5 ounces) puffed rice cereal	12
with ¼ cup Almond Milk	2
1 cup herbal tea	0

DAY 4 (continued)

LUNCH

Savory Spanish Salad	11
Savory Spanish Dressing	6
1 rice cake	8
Spring or mineral water	0

DINNER

Chicken Cutlets Italiano	25
Spinach and Egg Salad	7
2 tablespoons Avocado and Lemon-Herb Dressing	0

SNACK

1 cup popcorn, popped	4
with Easy Clarified Butter	0
TOTAL CARBOHYDRATES	75

DAY 5

	Carbohydrate Grams
BREAKFAST	
1 Oat and Orange Muffin	15
1 cup herbal tea	0
LUNCH	
Cantonese Chicken Salad	5
1 rice cake	8
Spring or mineral water	0
DINNER	
Florentine-Stuffed Sole	6
Delicious Lokchen Kugel	33
Fancy Red and Green Slaw	7
½ cup scrubbed and sliced zucchini, cooked	2
SNACK	
5 rice crackers	7
TOTAL CARBOHYDRATES	83

DAY 6

	Carbohydrate Grams
BREAKFAST	
California Omelet	10
1 cup Taheebo Tea (optional)	0
LUNCH	
1 Greek-Style Breast of Chicken	3
1 rice cake	8
1 medium fresh tomato, scrubbed and sliced	4
Spring or mineral water	0
DINNER	
Linguini with Clams and Garlic Sauce	22
½ cup cooked frozen spinach	4
1 cup scrubbed and shredded lettuce	2
2 tablespoons Thousand Island Dressing	1
SNACK	
1 Sunny Corn Muffin	23
with Easy Clarified Butter	0
TOTAL CARBOHYDRATES	77

DAY 7

	Carbohydrate Grams
BREAKFAST	
1 mochi (Japanese rice cake)	34
Easy Clarified Butter	0
1 cup herbal tea	0
LUNCH	
Delicious Shrimp Louis	5
1 rice cake	8
Spring or mineral water	0

DAY 7 *(continued)*

DINNER

Marinated and Stuffed Flank Steak	8
½ cup scrubbed and sliced zucchini, cooked	2
Spinach and Egg Salad	7
2 tablespoons Avocado and Lemon-Herb Dressing	0

SNACK

1 cup plain nonfat yogurt, sweetened	6
with 100% Pure Vegetable Glycerine	0
TOTAL CARBOHYDRATES	70

DAY 8

	Carbohydrate Grams
BREAKFAST	
1 Sunny Corn Muffin	23
1 cup Taheebo Tea (optional)	0
LUNCH	
Shrimp-Topped Rice Cake	10
Cranberry Zinger	9
DINNER	
Chicken Cacciatore	5
Special Lemon Rice	22
½ cup scrubbed and chopped asparagus, freshly cooked	3
1 cup iced herbal tea	0
SNACK	
1 rice cake	8
TOTAL CARBOHYDRATES	80

DAY 9

	Carbohydrate Grams
BREAKFAST	
Scrambled Eggs with a Flair	5
1 cup Taheebo Tea (optional)	0
LUNCH	
1 Florentine-Stuffed Tomato	14
1 rice cake	8
Spring or mineral water with fresh lime	0
DINNER	
Tomato and Beef Soup with Brown Rice	24
Eggplant Supreme	18
Delightful Cheesecake	9
SNACK	
5 brown rice crackers	7
TOTAL CARBOHYDRATES	85

DAY 10

	Carbohydrate Grams
BREAKFAST	
1 poached egg	1
1 rice cake	8
1 cup herbal tea	0
LUNCH	
Super Salmon Salad	20
Spring or mineral water	0

DAY 10 *(continued)*

DINNER

Lemon-Sautéed Chicken and Vegetables	13
½ cup cooked brown rice	25
Spinach and Egg Salad	7
2 tablespoons Basil and Garlic Salad Oil	2

SNACK

½ cup plain nonfat yogurt, sweetened	6
with 100% Pure Vegetable Glycerine	0
TOTAL CARBOHYDRATES	82

DAY 11

	Carbohydrate Grams
BREAKFAST	
1 heaping cup (5 ounces) puffed rice cereal	12
with ¼ cup Almond Milk	2
1 cup Taheebo Tea (optional)	0
LUNCH	
Shrimp-Stuffed Avocado	10
Spring or mineral water	0
DINNER	
Chicken-Kasha Soup	16
Veal Meatballs and Spaghetti	20
(1 ounce soba spaghetti)	12
½ cup cooked chopped broccoli	4
SNACK	
1 cup popcorn, popped	4
with Easy Clarified Butter	0
TOTAL CARBOHYDRATES	80

DAY 12

	Carbohydrate Grams
BREAKFAST	
Fiesta Frittata	13
1 cup Taheebo Tea	0
LUNCH	
Greek-Style Breast of Chicken	3
1 cup scrubbed and chopped fresh spinach	2
2 tablespoons Poppy Seed French Dressing	2
½ medium fresh tomato, scrubbed and sliced	2
Spring or mineral water with fresh lime	0
DINNER	
Shrimp and Rice Delight	33
1 Sunny Corn Muffin	23
SNACK	
1 rice cake	8
with Almond Butter	2
TOTAL CARBOHYDRATES	88

DAY 13

	Carbohydrate Grams
BREAKFAST	
1 Oat and Orange Muffin	15
1 cup Taheebo Tea (optional)	0
LUNCH	
1 Gourmet Tuna-Stuffed Tomato	11
Spring or mineral water with fresh lime	0

DAY 13 *(continued)*

DINNER

Meatballs with Sweet and Sour Sauce	16
1 ounce soba spaghetti	12
1 cup scrubbed and chopped lettuce	2
½ cup cucumber, scrubbed, peeled, and sliced	4
2 tablespoons Creamy Herb Dressing	2

SNACK

½ cup sliced fresh almonds (see note)	14
TOTAL CARBOHYDRATES	76

Note: If digestive system is sensitive, do not use nuts; 10 brown rice crackers may be used instead.

DAY 14

	Carbohydrate Grams
BREAKFAST	
1 Zucchini Frittata	9
1 rice cake	8
Easy Clarified Butter	0
1 cup herbal tea	0
LUNCH	
Marinated Buckwheat Salad	35
Spring or mineral water	0
DINNER	
Sautéed Sole Monterey	26
½ cup scrubbed and chopped fresh spinach	1
2 tablespoons Basil and Garlic Salad Oil	0
SNACK	
½ cup plain nonfat yogurt, sweetened	6
with 100% Pure Vegetable Glycerine	0
TOTAL CARBOHYDRATES	85

Carbohydrate Guide

A carbohydrate guide enables *Candida* patients to familiarize themselves with the amount of carbohydrates in permitted foods. This allows for easier planning of daily menus.

Note: The following carbohydrate information was obtained from *Nutritive Value of American Foods in Common Units*,*

Food	Carbohydrate Grams	Food	Carbohydrate Grams
Abalone	0	Baking powder	
Agar-Agar (seaweed		(1 teaspoon)	1
gelatin)	0	(1 tablespoon)	4
Albacore tuna	0	Bamboo shoots, raw	4
Almonds, fresh	14	Bass	2
Almonds, roasted	15	Bean flour, garbanzo	
Amaranth flour	70	(1 tablespoon)	4
Arrowroot powder		Bean flour, lima	
(1 tablespoon)	7	(1 tablespoon)	5
Artichoke (1 medium)	12	Beans, black, raw	61
Artichokes, Jerusalem		Beans, French, frozen	7
(4 miniature)	17	Beans, garbanzo	
Asparagus, cooked		(chick-peas)	61
(4 medium spears)	2	Beans, green, fresh,	
Asparagus, fresh	3	cooked	3
Avocado (1 medium)	13	Beans, green, fresh	4

*Agriculture Handbook #456, U.S. Department of Agriculture, 1975. The carbohydrate grams are based upon 4 ounces, unless otherwise shown.

Food	Carbohydrate Grams	Food	Carbohydrate Grams
Beans, kidney, cooked	20	Chestnuts, fresh	20
Beans, lima, cooked	17	Chicken	0
Beans, pinto	61	Chicken broth, Hain's.	
Beans, refried	20	unsweetened	2
Beef	0	Chicken liver (each)	2
Beets, raw (2 beets)	7	Chikory	1
Bifun		Chili pepper, small,	
(100% wheat-free		green (each)	7
Chinese noodles)	46	Chives (1 teaspoon)	1
Brazil nuts	8	Clams, canned	
Broccoli, frozen,		(unsweetened, no	
cooked	4	MSG)	3
Broccoli, raw	7	Clams, raw (4 or 5	
Broccoli, raw, cooked	4	clams)	4
Brown rice, cooked		Club soda	
(organic, preferably)	25	(unsweetened)	0
Brown rice, raw		Cod	0
(organic, preferably)	72	Corn, canned	
Brown rice crackers		(unsweetened)	9
(5 crackers)	7	Corn chips	60
Brown rice flour	88	Corn flour	45
Brussels sprouts,		Corn, fresh	16
cooked	5	Cornish hen	0
Buckwheat (1.3 ounces		Cornmeal	45
uncooked or		Corn noodles and	
¾ cup cooked)	30	spaghetti	88
Buckwheat flour, dark	35	Cornstarch	
Buckwheat flour, light	39	(1 tablespoon)	7
Butter, almond	14	Corn tortilla (each)	14
Butter, cashew	21	Cottage cheese, raw	4
Butter, clarified	0	Crab	0
Cabbage, cooked	3	Crackers, brown rice	
Cabbage, green, raw	4	(5 crackers)	7
Cabbage, red, raw	2	Cranberry concentrate	
Caraway seeds		(natural,	
(1 teaspoon)	1	unsweetened)	
Carrots,		(1 ounce, with	
raw (each)	7	water)	18
cooked (diced or		Cream of Rice Cereal	
sliced)	5	(1 ounce,	
Cashews	21	uncooked)	18
Caviar, sturgeon, granular		Crispy Cakes, natural	
(1 tablespoon)	1	(each)	4
Celery (1 stalk)	2	Crookneck squash,	
Cheese, raw cottage	4	yellow	3

Food	Carbohydrate Grams	Food	Carbohydrate Grams
Cucumber, pared and sliced		Lima beans	17
		Lime (medium)	6
(1 small)	5	Lime juice, fresh	11
(1 large)	9	Liver, beef	6
Delicious Homemade		Liver, chicken	4
Mayonnaise	2	Lobster	0
Egg		Lychees, raw	
(large, raw)	1	(10 lychees)	15
(medium, raw)	0	Macadamia nuts	18
Eggplant	4	Mayonnaise,	
Endive	1	Delicious	
Escarole	1	Homemade	2
Filbert nuts (10 nuts)	2	Milk, Almond	14
Flounder	0	Milk, Cashew	21
Frog legs	0	Milk, soy	16
Garbanzo beans, fresh, cooked		Millet flour	42
		Mochi, plain	
(chick-peas)	61	(each square)	34
Garbanzo flour	31	Noodles, corn (corn	
Garlic, peeled		ribbons, etc.)	88
(1 clove)	1	Nuts, almond (4 oz)	14
Gelatin, plain	0	Nuts, Brazil (4 oz)	8
Goose	0	Nuts, cashew (4 oz)	21
Grits	63	Nuts, lychee (10	
Haddock	7	lychees)	15
Halibut	0	Nuts, pecan (4 oz)	8
Hazelnuts (10 nuts)	2	Nuts, walnut (4 oz)	10
Hickory nuts	14	Oat bran (1/3 cup raw)	17
Jerusalem artichokes		Oats (1/3 cup raw)	16
(4 artichokes)	17	Oils, olive, safflower,	
Jicama	N/A	sesame	0
Kale, cooked	3	Okra, cooked	5
Kasha (buckwheat), (1.3 ounces uncooked		Olives, ripe, sliced	
or ¾ cup cooked)	30	(canned) (per 4 oz)	2
Lamb	0	Onion, medium, yellow or white	
Leeks	13	(each or 1 cup)	14
Lemon (medium)	6	Onion, green (2 large	
Lemon juice, fresh		or 6 small)	3
(1 tablespoon)	1	Orange Roughy fish	0
Lemon peel		Oysters, fresh	4
(1 tablespoon)	1	Parsley	3
Lentils, cooked	20	Parsnips, cooked	12
Lettuce	1		
Lima bean flour, sifted	40		

Food	Carbohydrate Grams	Food	Carbohydrate Grams
Pea pods (snow peas or sugar peas), fresh, cooked	11	Red snapper	8
Pea pods, frozen	14	Rhubarb	2
Peas, fresh	11	Rice, brown, raw (organic, preferably)	72
Peas, fresh, cooked	10	cooked (organic, preferably)	25
Peas, frozen, cooked	9	Rice cakes (each)	8
Pecans	8	Rice Crackers (5 crackers)	7
Pepper, green bell, large (each)	8	Rice, Cream of, Cereal (1 ounce, uncooked)	23
Pepper, green bell, medium (each)	4	Rice flour, brown	88
Pepper, red bell, medium (each)	5	Rice, Puffed, Cereal (1 heaping cup or 5 ounces)	13
Perch	8	Rice and Shine Cereal (¼ cup, uncooked)	35
Perrier	0	Rice, wild, raw	60
Pheasant	0	Romaine lettuce	1
Pike	0	Rutabaga, cooked	7
Pine nuts, shelled	13	Salmon	0
Pinto beans	61	Scallops, cooked	0
Popcorn, popped, plain	2	Seltzer water	0
Poppyseeds (1 tablespoon)	3	Sesame seeds (1 teaspoon)	1
Pork	0	Shallots, raw (each tablespoon)	2
Potato, large, pared and boiled (each)	27	Shrimp, small	1
Potato, medium, pared and boiled (each)	16	Snow peas (pea pods or sugar peas)	11
Potato flour (1 tablespoon)	10	Soba (Japanese 100% buckwheat spaghetti)	46
Puffed Rice Cereal (1 heaping cup or 5 ounces)	12	Sole	0
Pumpkin, canned (unsweetened)	10	Soy flour	36
Quail	0	Soy milk	32
Quinoa (1 ounce dry or 4 ounces cooked)	18	Spaghetti, buckwheat (soba)	46
Quinoa flour (2 ounces)	35	Spaghetti, corn	88
Rabbit	0	Spinach, fresh	1
Radishes (10 medium)	2	Spinach, frozen, cooked	4
Raw cottage cheese	4		

Food	Carbohydrate Grams	Food	Carbohydrate Grams
Squash, crookneck, yellow	3	Tongue, beef	0
		Tortilla chips	24
Sunflower kernels (1 tablespoon)	2	Tortilla, corn (each)	14
		Tuna	0
Sweet potato, cooked (each)	37	Turkey, cooked	0
		Turnips, cooked	4
Swiss chard, cooked	2	Veal	0
Teas, herb	0	Vegetable Glycerine, 100% Pure (permitted sweetener)	0
Tofu	3		
Tomato, large, raw (each)	6		
(cooked, ½ cup)	7	Walnuts	10
Tomato (each, medium)	4	Water chestnuts	17
		Whitefish	0
Tomato, cherry, whole, fresh (4 tomatoes)	3	Wild rice, raw	60
		Yams	23
		Yogurt, plain, low-fat	6
Tomato paste, canned (no citric acid)	20	Yogurt, plain, nonfat	6
Tomato sauce, canned (unsweetened, no citric acid)	9	Zucchini, cooked (1 pound)	16
		Zucchini, raw	2

A Few Words
Before . . .

*C*andida sensitivity need not make mealtime difficult. Over the years I've developed many delicious recipes, all made with tasty substitutes for forbidden ingredients. With the help of these recipes, you'll be able to entertain and enjoy eating again. Enjoy!

General Tips

People with yeast conditions may also be sensitive to certain chemical additives, foods, even odors. I've taken this into account in preparing the recipes; most questionable ingredients are optional, or substitutes can be found. However, it may be to your benefit to select recipes according to your individual sensitivities.

As I've mentioned, it's generally best to keep your carbohydrate count between 60 and 100 grams daily in the beginning stages of treatment. As your condition improves, you may gradually add more. For each recipe, I've provided a carbohydrate count. Also, consult the Carbohydrate Guide (pages 21–25) and the 14-day *Candida* Control Menu Plan (pages 11–20) for help in planning.

A high-sugar, high-starch diet provides a perfect environment in which yeast can thrive. Overeating also promotes yeast growth, so eating in moderation is advised.

Readers who have symptoms of hypoglycemia (low blood sugar) should be especially careful with the carbohydrate level of the diet; those who lose too much weight on the diet may increase the use of complex carbohydrates. For example, 1 cup of any cooked whole grain or beans is equal to 40–50 grams of carbohydrates; a large, boiled, and pared potato equals 27 grams. However, hypoglycemics, as other *Candida* sufferers, should consult a health care professional to determine exactly how many grams of carbohydrates they're allowed.

Ingredients and Substitutes

Clarified butter is preferable to regular butter on the diet because the clarifying eliminates the milk sugar, which may encourage yeast growth. This butter may be purchased in some specialty food stores; however, it is expensive. Therefore, the Easy Clarified Butter recipe (p. 37) should be helpful to you. The use of **margarine** is not advised on the diet because of its processing and many chemical additives.

All cheese, including **cottage cheese,** as well as **sour cream, milk, and buttermilk** should be avoided. A good substitute for cottage cheese is **raw cottage cheese,** but if your digestive system is sensitive, omit it. **Soy milk** is a good substitute for pasteurized milk. However, if you're sensitive to soy, **nut milk or egg whites** may be used instead (see "Dairy Substitutes," pages 37–39).

Since wheat, barley, oat, and rye flours are not permitted, other **wheatless flours,** such as **millet, buckwheat, potato, rice, corn, garbanzo, soy** and **amaranth**, as well as **arrowroot powder** may be used not only in baked goods but as thickeners for gravies and sauces.

Delicious substitutes for wheat noodles are **corn noodles, bifun (Chinese noodles), and soba (100% pure buckwheat spaghetti).** Some grain recipes contain **quinoa** (pronounced keenwa). Quinoa contains more protein than any other grain and is easy to digest.

You may find it helpful to bake muffins ahead of time and freeze and use them as needed. Actually, a good general rule is to prepare the quantity of food you'll need for a particular meal and freeze any leftovers. Food begins to collect bacteria, which can be very harmful to your health, within 24 hours.

Rice cakes are good for snacking and as bread substitutes. Each cake has only 7–8 grams of carbohydrates and is very filling. They are especially delicious when spread with butters or popped into the microwave or oven to warm before eating. **Mochi**, a 2-inch-square rice cake that puffs up when baked, is another delicious breakfast and snack item. It can be eaten plain, spread with butters, or stuffed. A word of caution: Each mochi square contains 34 carbohydrates and is best to eat when other foods are low in carbohydrates.

It's preferable to heat foods in **100% pure cold-pressed olive oil** rather than other oils because its properties do not change when moderately heated and it can keep yeast from spreading further. It is also the best oil to use for salads.

100% Pure Vegetable Glycerine is a good substitute for other sweeteners. It is an excellent substitute in baking and cooking.

If you eat **tofu,** stick to what's very fresh, not stored.

For people sensitive to corn, **arrowroot powder** is a good substitute for **cornstarch** and is used in many recipes in this book.

If your digestive system is very sensitive, it's best to omit all nuts and seeds in beginning stages of the diet. Keep in mind that fresh nuts are preferable to others and the ground nuts are easier to digest than chopped.

Most commercially prepared extract flavorings—vanilla, almond, mint, and so on—contain alcohol and should be avoided. **Flavorings** containing no alcohol, sugar, or salt are available in many flavors in health and natural food stores.

Dining Out

Dining out need not be a difficult experience—it can even be enjoyable! You will find that restaurants are accommodating these days because many people are so diet conscious. Tell your waiter that you wish to:

- Have mineral water instead of wine
- Pass on the breadbasket (you can do it!)
- Avoid any entrées cooked with wine, sugar, flour, or milk; lemon, olive oil, and butter are okay
- Skip any gravies and mushrooms
- Have shrimp cocktail with lemon instead of sauce
- Eat your salad with lemon juice and oil
- Pass on the sour cream with your potato
- Savor herbal tea instead of dessert

Living on the Safe Side

Your doctor is likely to prescribe some antifungal agents to help your system deal with yeast overgrowth. The most common are **Nystatin, Nizoral**, and **Mycocidin**. There are also several nonprescription products, such as **biotin**, that may prove beneficial. Be sure to check with your doctor. There are several types of tests available that can confirm a *Candida* infection; be aware, however, that they must be administered by a health care professional.

Yeast is the basis for many vitamin and mineral preparations and should be avoided. **Tryptophan**, often used as a natural relaxant, is often derived from yeast. Check health and natural food stores for yeast-free supplements.

Yeasts also love an acid-free environment. Since all **prescription and nonprescription antacids** promote these conditions, they are to be avoided while you are on the treatment program. Instead, use **charcoal capsules or tablets** for stomach distress. **Hydrochloric acid capsules or tablets** if tolerable, aids in digestion, while its acidification lowers yeast. **Acidophilus** capsules, tablets, or powder places acid into your system, has flora-replacing bacteria properties, and is an immune system builder as well. **Bifidus** is very soothing and healing for stomach distress and diarrhea. **Aloe vera** liquid (pure only) used orally and topically, is also very soothing and healing. All of these supplements are available in health and natural food stores. **Appendix A, "Nutritional Supplements for the *Candida* Condition,"** will give you more information on them.

Before beginning this program, it is important to become as knowledgeable as possible about the things that can benefit your condition and those that can be detrimental. Please be certain to have a health care professional supervise your recovery.

Important Information on Recipe Ingredients

*T*here are many ingredients that are recommended for the *Candida* condition and many to avoid. Those recommended are usually not available in your grocery store, but are found in most health and natural food stores. If that specialty store does not carry the product, please refer to Appendix B for source information. The following products are alphabetized for your convenience:

Agar-Agar is a seaweed substitute for animal gelatin, and does not contain antibiotics or steroids that animal gelatin contains.

Arrowroot powder is a good cornstarch substitute or thickener for those sensitive to corn.

Beans that are raw should be washed thoroughly by placing them in a colander in your sink and running water over them several times.

Brown rice should be organic, short-grain preferably. However, long-grain is acceptable. Be certain not to purchase "instant brown rice" from your regular grocery store, as this product is sweetened and contains additives.

Brown rice chips/crackers should only be wheatless and without tamari, honey or fruit.

Cereals, dry or cooked, should not contain malt, honey or other sweeteners, fruit or yeast.

Cheese should contain no mold or citric acid and should be unsweetened. The only cheese this book recommends is raw cottage cheese, but it should be avoided if your digestive system is sensitive because it may be hard to digest. Do not purchase soy cheese. All have citric acid as well as additives that should be avoided.

Chicken broth should be unsweetened. Hain's makes both a sweetened and unsweetened chicken broth. Make certain that you purchase Hain's Naturals Home-Style Soup (the unsweetened one).

Corn should contain no sweeteners, preservatives or additives. There is a canned corn by Co-op, which is unsweetened, without preservatives and a frozen corn by Health Valley, that has no preservatives, chemicals or pesticides. *Beware, though: Many people are sensitive to corn.*

Cranberry concentrate, is recommended because it is pure, unsweetened and low in carbohydrates.

Flavorings should not contain alcohol, sugar or salt. Many flavors, which meet those requirements, are available in most health and natural food stores.

Flours should only be wheatless and without gluten. Those recommended are amaranth, buckwheat, corn, garbanzo, millet, potato, rice and soy flours. Also quinoa flour is a fairly new and good one.

Meats and **Poultry** should be naturally grown, without growth hormones, steroids or antibiotics. To make certain, check with the producer instead of your butcher.

Noodles should be wheat-free. Read your labels carefully. The recommended noodles are:
  Bifun (100% wheat-free Chinese noodles)
  DeBoles Corn Ribbons (and other corn noodles and spaghetti)
  Harasume (Japanese rice noodles)
  Kuzu-Kiri (Japanese clear noodles)
  Soba (100% pure buckwheat Japanese noodles)

Nuts and seeds may be difficult on your digestive system in the beginning stages of treatment. Ground nuts are easier to digest than chopped or you may be wise to omit nuts and seeds until your condition improves.

Olive oil should be 100% pure, cold-pressed or expeller-pressed. It is beneficial for *Candida* conditions because it doesn't lose its properties when heated and is delicious in salad dressings and marinades.

Quinoa, pronounced keenwa, is a substitute for wheat. It is mother grain, contains more protein than any other grain and is easy to digest.

Rice cakes, made with brown rice, should be unsweetened and without tamari.

Safflower oil should be 100% pure, cold-pressed or expeller-pressed. Don't use coconut, corn, cottonseed peanut or vegetable oils.

Sea salt should be free of additives and sweeteners. La Baleine Sea Salt accomplishes this. Don't use regular table salt; it contains additives and dextrose.

Soy milk should be pure and natural. Be certain that you aren't sensitive to soy, and don't purchase any that contain malt, flavorings, honey or other sweeteners.

Taheebo Tea (also known as La Pacho, Ipe Roxo, Tabeuia, Tecoma, Bow Stick), a tea grown in the rain forests of South America, is free of fungus and can be beneficial in the treatment of *Candida*. Some people cannot tolerate the tea, so I recommend that you try it in small amounts and increase it gradually.

Tofu should be fresh and not stored. Check the date with your produce supplier.

Tomatoes should be fresh. If you wish to use tomatoes for cooking, first scrub them. Then peel, core, purée or chop and strain, if necessary. *Do not buy canned tomatoes.* They all contain citric acid and other preservatives and additives.

Tomato sauce should be unsweetened and contain no citric acid

Vegetable Glycerine, by Herbcraft, is a permitted sweetener. It is 100% pure, contains no carbohydrates nor cholesterol. Derived from coconut oil, this product is excellent in baking and cooking. One tablespoon of this glycerine is equivalent to approximately 1/4 cup of sugar. However, when the glycerine is heated, some of its flavor evaporates, so you may wish to use a little more. It is best to mix it into sauces after they have cooked.

Vegetables should usually be fresh. If using fresh vegetables, be sure to scrub them to avoid digesting mold. There are some recipes in this book that use frozen vegetables such as broccoli and spinach. Health Valley Natural Foods sells vegetables that are unsweetened and contain no preservatives, additives or pesticides. Do not use any other frozen vegetables unless they meet these specifications.

Water should be purified because of chemical sensitivities.

Yogurt may be purchased in your grocery store if it is natural, without fruit, honey or other sweeteners, preservatives or additives.

Please be aware that if you have *Candida,* you probably also have a sensitive digestive system and/or have sensitivities to many foods, additives, and preservatives. Therefore, do try to follow the many suggestions that have been given in this section. It is important to rotate your foods, to introduce one new one at a time and to eat in moderate amounts. Remember, also, to read all labels carefully. The best way that you can conquer *Candida,* in addition to your treatment program, is to be knowledgeable about problem foods and permitted foods and then to be conscientious and consistent with the diet program.

Dairy Substitutes

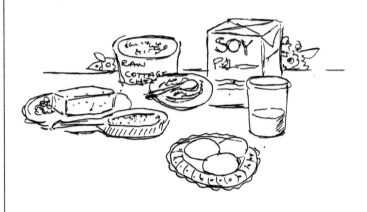

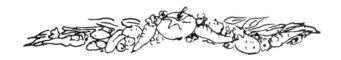

Delicious and Easy Nut Butter

YIELDS APPROXIMATELY ½ CUP

½ cup fresh raw pecans,   *1 tablespoon safflower oil*
walnuts, or almonds

Combine nuts and oil in a food processor or blender; mix until creamy. Spread on rice cakes or rice crackers or use in recipes.

Almond butter = 14 carbohydrates; 1 tablespoon = 2
Pecan butter = 8 carbohydrates; 1 tablespoon = 1
Walnut butter = 9 carbohydrates; 1 tablespoon = 1

Easy Clarified Butter

YIELDS ½ CUP OR MORE

Clarifying butter is recommended because it eliminates the milk sugar that may be harmful for a *Candida* or yeast condition. A good amount of butter may be clarified at one time and stored for later use.

½ cup to 1 pound unsalted butter

Skillet Method

Heat amount of butter desired in a small skillet. When melted and completely separated, skim off the white residue (milk sugar) from the top; discard. Pour the clear yellow liquid into a storage container; discard residue on bottom of skillet. When cool, cover storage container with a tight-fitting lid.

Microwave Method

Cut amount of butter desired into ¼-inch squares; place them in a microwave-safe container. Heat on medium-high for just a few seconds or until the butter melts and becomes completely separated. Skim off white residue from top; discard. Pour the clear yellow liquid into a storage container; discard residue on bottom of microwave container. When cool, cover storage container with a tight-fitting lid.

0 carbohydrates

Note: Refrigerate clarified butter.

Almond Milk

YIELDS APPROXIMATELY 1 QUART OR MORE

This is a delicious alternative to pasteurized or soy milk.

1 cup fresh raw almonds
2 cups boiling water (purified, preferably)
1 quart cold water (purified, preferably)

1 tablespoon pure, cold-pressed safflower oil
2 tablespoons 100% Pure Vegetable Glycerine
¼ teaspoon sea salt (optional)

Blanch almonds by pouring boiling water over nuts; soak a few minutes or until skins slide off easily; drain. Place skinless almonds, cold water, oil, glycerine, and salt in a food processor or blender. Process to a very smooth liquid. If necessary, strain with cheesecloth or a fine strainer; refrigerate. Use in recipes as you would pasteurized or soy milk.

4 carbohydrates per ½ cup

Cashew Milk

YIELDS APPROXIMATELY 1 QUART OR MORE

This is an easy-to-prepare alternative to pasteurized or soy milk.

1 cup fresh raw cashews
1 quart cold water (purified, preferably)
1 tablespoon pure, cold-pressed safflower oil

2 tablespoons 100% Pure Vegetable Glycerine
¼ teaspoon sea salt (optional)

Place all ingredients in a food processor or blender. Process to a very smooth liquid. If necessary, strain with cheesecloth or a fine strainer; refrigerate. Use in recipes as you would pasteurized or soy milk.

4 carbohydrates per ½ cup

Egg Whites as a Milk Substitute

1 BEATEN LARGE EGG WHITE = ½–1 CUP MILK
2 BEATEN LARGE EGG WHITES = 1½–2 CUPS MILK
3 BEATEN LARGE EGG WHITES = 2½–3 CUPS MILK

If you're sensitive to soy or nut milk, egg whites are a wonderful alternative—and are very easy to prepare.

Beat egg whites in a mixing bowl with electric mixer or food processor until creamy (but not stiff) and use as you would milk.

0 carbohydrates

Mock Sour Cream

YIELDS APPROXIMATELY 1 CUP

Yogurt and glycerine make a delicious substitution for sour cream.

1 cup plain low-fat yogurt   *1 teaspoon 100% Pure Vegetable Glycerine*

Mix yogurt and glycerine in a small bowl. Chill at least 30 minutes before serving.

12 carbohydrates

Appetizers and Hors d'Oeuvres

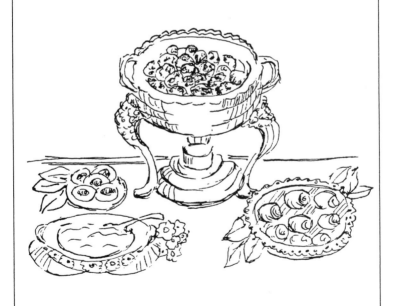

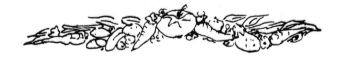

Caviar and Eggs

YIELDS 6 SERVINGS

This is a very elegant and delicious appetizer to serve guests. Expect many compliments!

6 large eggs, hard-cooked, cooled, and peeled
2 tablespoons scrubbed, peeled, and chopped yellow onion
2 tablespoons Delicious Home-made Mayonnaise (page 145)

2 tablespoons plain low-fat yogurt (see note)
1 jar (2.1 ounces) lumpfish caviar (see note)
Fresh parsley sprigs for garnish
Brown rice crackers

Place eggs in a food processor and chop, or chop by hand. Spoon mixture into a small bowl. Add onion and mayonnaise; mix. Refrigerate for at least 1 hour before serving. Remove from refrigerator; turn bowl upside down on the center of a large round serving plate. Cover mound with yogurt; spoon caviar over top. Garnish with parsley; surround with rice crackers.

1 carbohydrate per serving

Note: If your digestive system is sensitive, omit yogurt and make the egg mixture creamier. Cooked baby shrimp may be used instead of caviar if you wish.

Chicken Pâté

YIELDS 4 TO 6 SERVINGS

This is a delightful pâté for any occasion; it can even be molded into shapes to suit any occasion.

*2 tablespoons melted chicken
  fat or Easy Clarified Butter
  (page 37)*
4 chicken livers, cleaned
*1 medium yellow onion,
  scrubbed, peeled, and sliced*

*2 large eggs, hard-cooked,
  cooled, and peeled*
½ teaspoon sea salt (optional)
Fresh parsley sprigs for garnish
Brown rice crackers

Heat fat or butter; sauté livers and onion until browned. Grate liver, onion, and eggs in a food processor, grinder, or blender until you've achieved a thick, smooth consistency; add salt. Place pâté in a small bowl or greased mold. Cover and refrigerate for 1 hour to allow flavors to blend before serving. Garnish with parsley; serve with brown rice crackers.

6 carbohydrates per serving for 4; 4 carbohydrates per serving for 6

Chicken Wings

YIELDS 16 WINGS

This is an easy, scrumptious appetizer that everyone will enjoy.

16 chicken wings
*⅓ cup Easy Clarified Butter
  (page 37)*

¾ cup brown rice flour
½ teaspoon sea salt (optional)
1 teaspoon garlic powder

Preheat oven to 400°F. Cut and discard wing tips. Melt butter in a small skillet. Remove from heat. Place flour and seasonings in a shallow dish; mix. Dip wings into butter, then into the flour mixture; turn into a large baking dish. Bake 20 minutes; turn. Bake 20 minutes longer, or until golden brown.

8 carbohydrates each

La Favorita Guacamole

YIELDS 4 TO 6 SERVINGS

This delicious guacamole is served in a tortilla bowl!

1 medium avocado, scrubbed,
peeled, pitted, and grated
2 tablespoons fresh lemon juice
1 large fresh tomato, scrubbed
and chopped

3 small green onions, scrubbed,
peeled, and chopped
½ teaspoon garlic powder
Cayenne pepper to taste

Combine avocado and lemon juice in a food processor or blender; mix until creamy. Place in a small bowl. Add tomato, onions, and seasonings; mix. Place into Mexican Tortilla Bowl (below).

2 to 4 carbohydrates per serving

Mexican Tortilla Bowl

100% pure, cold-pressed olive oil
1 corn tortilla

Tortilla chips

Cover bottom of a small skillet with oil; when hot, add tortilla. Heat just until tortilla bubbles and lifts. Turn with tongs; repeat process on other side. Blot and quickly place in a small bowl. Press against sides; let set 5–10 minutes. Place tortilla bowl on a serving plate; fill with guacamole. Surround with chips.

Tortilla = 14 carbohydrates; chips = 6 carbohydrates per ounce

Party-Stuffed Eggs

YIELDS 1 DOZEN STUFFED EGG HALVES

For a fancy appetizer, this is an excellent choice—and the cayenne is good for digestion.

6 large eggs, hard-cooked,
  cooled, and peeled
2 tablespoons Delicious Home-
  made Mayonnaise (page 145)
1 tablespoon chopped fresh basil

½ teaspoon garlic powder
¼ pound cooked baby shrimp,
  rinsed and chopped
Dash cayenne pepper
Fresh parsley sprigs for garnish

Cut each egg in half lengthwise. Scoop out yolk; mix yolks in a food processor or with fork until smooth. Blend in mayonnaise and seasonings. Gently fold in shrimp. Spoon mixture into egg white cavities. Sprinkle cayenne pepper lightly over tops. Garnish with parsley sprigs.

0 carbohydrates

Shrimp-Stuffed Cherry Tomatoes

YIELDS 1 DOZEN STUFFED CHERRY TOMATOES

These stuffed cherry tomatoes make elegant and tasty appetizers. There won't be any leftovers!

⅓ pound cooked baby shrimp,
  rinsed
1 stalk celery, scrubbed and finely
  chopped
½ teaspoon chopped fresh basil
½ teaspoon garlic powder

2 tablespoons Delicious Home-
  made Mayonnaise (page 145)
1 dozen cherry tomatoes,
  scrubbed, pulp removed
Fresh parsley sprigs for garnish

Combine shrimp, celery, basil, garlic powder, and mayonnaise in a small mixing bowl; mix. Place tomatoes on a serving platter; stuff with filling. Place parsley sprigs between and around tomatoes to garnish. Chill 1–2 hours before serving to allow flavors to blend.

1 carbohydrate each

Turkey Roll-Ups
YIELDS APPROXIMATELY 1 DOZEN

A delicious alternative to bread appetizers!

*½ cup Delicious Homemade
   Mayonnaise (page 145)*
*2 stalks celery (without leaves),
   finely chopped*
¼ cup ground fresh walnuts

*1 tablespoon each chopped fresh
   basil and parsley*
*6 large slices cooked natural
   turkey*
Fresh parsley sprigs

Spoon mayonnaise into a small bowl. Add celery, walnuts and seasonings; mix. Spread evenly over top of turkey slices. Roll each slice tightly; cut in half. Place on a serving platter; garnish with parsley.

1 carbohydrate each

Soups

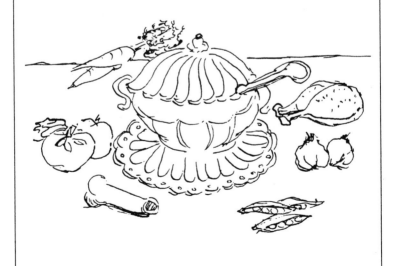

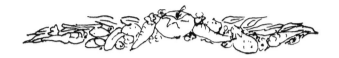

Best Clam Chowder

YIELDS 4 SERVINGS

Fresh tomatoes make for an easy and tasty chowder.

2 large fresh tomatoes, scrubbed, peeled, cored, puréed, and strained
1 cup water (purified, preferably)
1 can (6½ ounces) unsweetened minced clams (without MSG), undrained
1 medium new potato, scrubbed, peeled, and diced
1 medium red bell pepper, scrubbed and diced

1 medium yellow onion, scrubbed, peeled, and finely chopped
1 large clove garlic, scrubbed, peeled, and minced
1 tablespoon each chopped fresh parsley, sage, and thyme
¼ teaspoon ground nutmeg

Combine all ingredients in a large kettle; mix and bring to a boil. Reduce heat; cover and simmer 15 minutes, or until potato and vegetables are tender.

14 carbohydrates per serving

Chicken–Egg Drop Soup with Lemon

YIELDS 6 SERVINGS

This soup is extremely low in carbohydrates. Fresh lemon juice gives it a delightful flavor.

*1 frying chicken (approximately
  3 pounds), quartered
Water (purified, preferably)
1 medium yellow onion,
  scrubbed, peeled, and coarsely
  chopped*

*Sea salt to taste (optional)
1 teaspoon ground nutmeg
½ cup fresh lemon juice
2 large eggs, beaten*

Place chicken in a large kettle; add water to cover and bring to a boil. Reduce heat; add onion, salt, and nutmeg. Cover; simmer 1 hour. Remove chicken, reserving broth. Cool; remove and discard skin and bones; dice chicken meat. Skim any fat off soup; add chicken and lemon juice. Return broth to heat. Using a teaspoon, drizzle egg into the soup. Serve immediately.

4 carbohydrates per serving

Chicken-Kasha Soup

YIELDS 6 SERVINGS

Kasha—roasted buckwheat groats—is a delicious substitute for noodles or rice and is perfect in combination with my mother's marvelous soup recipe.

*1 chicken (approximately 3
  pounds), cut into eighths
Water (purified, preferably)
1 medium yellow onion,
  scrubbed, peeled, and coarsely
  chopped
2 stalks celery, including leaves,
  scrubbed and chopped*

*2 cups scrubbed, peeled, and
  diced carrots
Garlic powder to taste
Sea salt to taste (optional)
1½ cups cooked kasha*

Place chicken in a large kettle; cover with water; bring to a boil. Skim off any foamy substance; reduce heat. Add vegetables and seasonings. Cover; simmer 1 hour. While the soup is cooking, prepare kasha according to package directions. Add to soup; heat for 10 minutes before serving. If you wish, remove chicken from soup and serve as a main dish.

16 carbohydrates per serving

Iced Gazpacho
YIELDS 4 SERVINGS

How refreshing to have this savory, icy soup on a hot day!

4 large fresh tomatoes, scrubbed, peeled, puréed and strained
1 medium yellow onion, scrubbed, peeled, and coarsely chopped
1 large clove garlic, minced
1 medium cucumber, scrubbed, peeled, and coarsely chopped
1 medium green bell pepper, scrubbed and coarsely chopped
2 stalks celery, without leaves, scrubbed and chopped
2 tablespoons fresh lemon juice
2 tablespoons chopped fresh basil
Cayenne pepper to taste
Sea salt to taste (optional)

Place all ingredients in a large mixing bowl; blend. Freeze bowl mixture 30 minutes, or until slushy. Serve immediately.

14 carbohydrates per serving

Oriental Chicken Noodle Soup

YIELDS 6 SERVINGS

Delicious bifun—Chinese wheat-free noodles—and fresh, savory seasonings make a delightful soup.

1½ frying chickens (approximately 4½ pounds), quartered
Water (purified, preferably)
1 medium yellow onion, scrubbed, peeled, and coarsely chopped
2 stalks celery, including leaves, scrubbed and chopped

2 large cloves garlic, scrubbed, peeled, and minced
2 tablespoons coarsely chopped fresh parsley
1 teaspoon each grated fresh ginger and nutmeg
½ package (2½ ounces) cooked and drained bifun

Place chickens in a large kettle. Cover with water; bring to a boil. Skim off any foamy substance. Add vegetables and seasonings. Reduce heat; cover and simmer 1 hour, or until chicken is tender. Remove chicken and serve separately if you wish. Skim off fat; add cooked noodles; mix and serve.

8 carbohydrates per serving

Savory Black Bean Soup

YIELDS 6 SERVINGS

This is a delicious, hearty soup for a cold day.

1 cup raw black beans, washed thoroughly soaked overnight, and drained
Water (purified, preferably)
1 tablespoon coarsely chopped fresh parsley
¾ teaspoon ground turmeric
⅛ teaspoon ground cumin
1 teaspoon each chopped fresh marjoram and thyme
2 tablespoons 100% pure, cold-pressed olive oil

2 large cloves garlic, scrubbed, peeled, and minced
1 medium yellow onion, scrubbed, peeled, and finely chopped
2 stalks celery, without leaves, scrubbed and finely chopped
1 can (6 ounces) tomato paste (without citric acid)
Sea salt to taste (optional)

Place beans in a large kettle; cover with water. Bring to a boil; cook 2 minutes; drain. Repeat process twice more. Place 1 quart water, beans, spices, and herbs in kettle; bring to a boil. Simmer, uncovered, 30 minutes. Spoon beans and their liquid into blender; blend until creamy. Place mixture in kettle; bring to a boil; simmer, uncovered. Heat oil in a small skillet. Sauté garlic and onion until tender; add, with tomato paste, to beans. Mix; cook uncovered 10 minutes and serve.

29 carbohydrates per serving

Simply Delicious and Easy Chicken Soup
YIELDS 4 SERVINGS

The title describes this soup perfectly. Enjoy!

1 pound chicken wings, cleaned
1 can (17½ ounces) unsweetened
  chicken broth
3 cups water (purified, preferably)
1 medium yellow onion,
  scrubbed, peeled, and coarsely
  chopped

1 large carrot, scrubbed, peeled,
  and cut into ¼ inch rounds
1 stalk celery including leaves,
  scrubbed and diced
¼ teaspoon sea salt (optional)
½ teaspoon ground nutmeg
¼ cup raw brown rice

Place wings, broth, and water in a 2-quart saucepan; bring to a boil and skim off any foamy substance. Reduce heat; add vegetables, seasonings, and rice. Cover; simmer 45 minutes, or until chicken is tender. Remove wings and serve separately or chill and use for chicken salad.

17 carbohydrates per serving

Tomato and Beef Soup with Brown Rice

YIELDS 4 SERVINGS

A wonderful, hearty soup for a cold day. Beef may be omitted if desired; soup will still be delicious!

2 large fresh tomatoes, scrubbed, peeled, and coarsely chopped
2 cups water (purified, preferably)
2 beef short ribs (approximately 1 pound total)
1 medium yellow onion, scrubbed, peeled, and diced
2 stalks celery, without leaves, scrubbed and thinly sliced
1 cup scrubbed and diced zucchini

½ teaspoon sea salt (optional)
1 teaspoon each chopped fresh sage, basil, and savory
2 tablespoons chopped fresh parsley
2 to 4 tablespoons chopped fresh cilantro, to taste
Garlic powder to taste
¼ cup raw brown rice

Combine tomatoes and water in a large kettle. Trim excess fat from ribs. Add ribs and rest of ingredients, including rice, to tomato mixture. Bring to a boil; reduce heat, cover, and simmer 1 hour. Skim off fat before serving.

18 carbohydrates per serving

Eggs

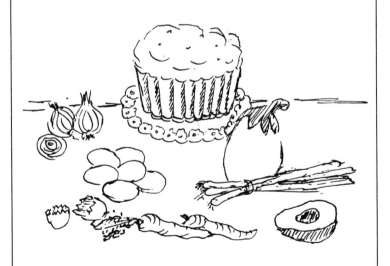

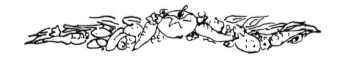

California Omelet

YIELDS 2 SERVINGS

A delicious idea for breakfast, lunch, or dinner.

4 large eggs
1 large tomato, scrubbed and diced
1 medium avocado, scrubbed, peeled, and diced
2 large green onions, scrubbed, peeled, and coarsely chopped

1 can (2.2 ounces) sliced ripe olives, drained (optional)
2 tablespoons Easy Clarified Butter (page 37)

Beat eggs in a medium bowl with a rotary beater or electric mixer. Add other ingredients, except butter; mix. Place butter in a large skillet; melt, moving pan back and forth until entire surface and sides are coated. Add egg mixture; cook over medium heat until sides and bottom are golden brown. Turn half of omelet over other half; cover. Cook at low heat until egg is set and omelet is golden brown.

10 carbohydrates per serving

Eggplant Frittata

YIELDS 4 SERVINGS

This delicious and elegant frittata may be served as a breakfast, lunch, or dinner entrée.

1 unpeeled eggplant (approximately 1¼ pounds), scrubbed
6 large eggs
2 tablespoons 100% pure, cold-pressed olive oil
3 large green onions, scrubbed, peeled, and coarsely chopped

1 medium red bell pepper, scrubbed and coarsely chopped
1 tablespoon chopped fresh basil
Sea salt to taste (optional)
Fresh basil sprigs for garnish

Cut eggplant in half. Scoop out edible fruit and cut it into bite-size chunks. Beat eggs in a large bowl. Add eggplant chunks to beaten eggs; soak 5 minutes. Heat oil in a large nonstick skillet. Add eggplant egg mixture, onion, red pepper, basil, and salt. Cook, covered, over medium-low heat until egg sets. Serve either hot or chilled. Garnish with basil sprigs.

8 carbohydrates per serving

Elegant Soufflé

YIELDS 6 SERVINGS

This is not only elegant but delicious as well.

2 tablespoons Easy Clarified Butter (page 37)
2 tablespoons brown rice flour
½ teaspoon sea salt (optional)

2 cups unsweetened soy milk (see note)
6 large eggs
1 teaspoon ground nutmeg

Preheat oven to 325°F. Melt butter in a 2-quart nonstick saucepan; stir in flour and salt. Add milk gradually; bring to a boil, stirring constantly. Reduce heat; simmer 2 minutes. Remove from heat; cool. Separate eggs; beat yolks into sauce. Beat whites until stiff; fold into sauce. Spoon mixture into a greased 10-inch casserole dish. Bake, uncovered, 1 hour, keeping oven door closed. Soufflé should be done when it is raised and golden brown. Sprinkle nutmeg over soufflé. Serve immediately.

26 carbohydrates per serving

Note: Try nut milk or egg white if you're sensitive to soy (see "Dairy Substitutes").

Fiesta Frittata

YIELDS 4 SERVINGS

This festive dish is a real delight for brunch guests.

4 large eggs
1 large tomato, scrubbed and
  diced
1 medium avocado, scrubbed,
  peeled, and diced
1 small fresh chili pepper,
  scrubbed and chopped

2 medium green onions,
  scrubbed, peeled, and chopped
100% pure, cold-pressed olive oil
2 corn tortillas
1 can (2.2 ounces) sliced ripe
  olives, drained (optional)
Saucy Salsa (page 179)

Beat eggs in a medium bowl. Add tomato, avocado, chili pepper, and onions; mix. Heat 2 tablespoons oil in a large, nonstick skillet. Pour egg mixture into same skillet. Cover, reduce heat to simmer. Eggs should cook 5–10 minutes longer or until they are set. Pour enough oil into another large skillet to cover the bottom. When oil is hot, heat tortillas just until they rise and begin to bubble; turn. When other side has risen, remove to a plate lined with paper towels. Cut each tortilla into 4 wedges. Surround top of egg frittata with tortilla wedges; garnish with olives. Serve with Saucy Salsa.

13 carbohydrates per serving

Scrambled Eggs with a Flair

YIELDS 4 SERVINGS

If you're tired of the same old way of preparing eggs, try this one!

8 large eggs
½ pound cooked baby shrimp, rinsed (see note)
1 medium avocado, scrubbed, peeled, and diced
1 medium red bell pepper, scrubbed and diced

2 medium green onions, scrubbed and diced
½ teaspoon garlic powder
Cayenne pepper to taste
2 tablespoons Easy Clarified Butter (page 37)
Fresh parsley sprigs for garnish

Beat eggs in a large bowl until light. Add rest of ingredients, except butter and parsley; mix. Melt butter in a large nonstick skillet. Pour egg mixture into skillet. Cook over medium-high heat, stirring frequently, until egg is set. Immediately transfer mixture to a serving platter; garnish with fresh parsley sprigs and serve.

5 carbohydrates per serving

Note: Crab may be used instead of shrimp if you wish.

Zucchini Frittata

YIELDS 4 SERVINGS

This is a favorite—for breakfast, lunch, or dinner.

6 large eggs
2 cups scrubbed and diced
*   zucchini*
1 medium yellow onion,
*   scrubbed, peeled, and chopped*
2 large cloves garlic, scrubbed,
*   peeled, and minced*

¼ cup chopped fresh parsley
Sea salt to taste (optional)
2 tablespoons 100% pure, cold-
*   pressed olive oil*

Beat eggs in a large bowl; add rest of ingredients, except oil, and mix. Heat oil in a large skillet; add egg mixture. Cook over medium-high heat until golden brown on bottom; turn and cook other side until egg is set.

9 carbohydrates per serving

Fish and Shellfish

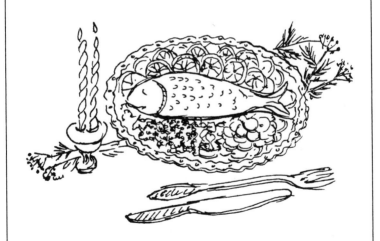

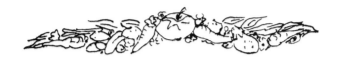

Deep-Fried Scallops

YIELDS 2 SERVINGS

This is an easy and quick recipe. Tasty Tartar Sauce (page 180) is a perfect accompaniment.

1 large egg
¼ cup brown rice flour
1 teaspoon garlic powder
1 teaspoon each chopped fresh basil and oregano

12 to 14 large scallops, cleaned
¾ cup 100% pure, cold-pressed olive oil
½ medium lemon, scrubbed and cut into wedges

Place egg into a small bowl; beat. Mix flour and seasonings in a small bowl. Rinse and dry scallops with paper towels. Pour oil into a nonstick skillet or wok; heat over medium-high heat. Dip each scallop first into egg, next into flour mixture, and then drop into hot oil for two minutes or until brown. When brown on one side, turn; brown other side. Place scallops on a plate lined with paper towels to drain. Serve with lemon wedges.

23 carbohydrates per serving

Elegant Foiled Red Snapper

YIELDS 4 SERVINGS

Other fish, such as bass, butterfish, orange roughy, salmon, or sole, may be prepared in the same manner.

4 red snapper fillets (approxi-
mately 8 ounces each)
Tasty Tartar Sauce (page 180)
¼ cup scrubbed and chopped
fresh broccoli florets
1 teaspoon chopped fresh dillweed

1 medium red bell pepper,
scrubbed and chopped
Cayenne pepper
1 medium lemon, scrubbed and
cut into thin rounds
Fresh parsley sprigs

Preheat oven to 350°F. Place each fillet on a 12-inch piece of foil. Mix tartar sauce, broccoli, dill and bell pepper in a small bowl. Spoon mixture, evenly divided, on each fillet; smooth over entire surface. Sprinkle cayenne lightly over each, then place lemon rounds and parsley sprigs over tops. Fold foil over fillets, rolling and sealing edges together. Place packets in a baking pan. Bake 20 minutes, or until fish flakes easily with a fork. Or barbecue if you like.

22 carbohydrates per serving

Fillet of Sole with Shrimp Stuffing

YIELDS 4 SERVINGS

This is an elegant and delicious way to prepare sole. Crab may be used instead of shrimp if you wish.

½ cup Easy Clarified Butter
(page 37) or 100% pure, cold-
pressed olive oil
1 teaspoon garlic powder
1 teaspoon each chopped fresh
basil and oregano
½ pound cooked baby shrimp,
rinsed

4 sole fillets (6 to 8 ounces each)
2 ounces fresh raw almonds,
sliced or ground (see note)
1 medium lemon, scrubbed and
sliced, for garnish
Fresh parsley sprigs for garnish

Preheat oven to 350°F. Melt butter in a large nonstick skillet. Add seasonings and shrimp; mix and remove from heat. Place shrimp mixture on the center of each fillet; reserve butter sauce in skillet. Roll fillets; secure with toothpicks. Place fillets in a greased 8-inch baking dish. Mix almonds into butter sauce; sprinkle over tops of fillets. Bake 20 minutes, or until fish flakes easily with a fork. Garnish with lemon and parsley.

2 carbohydrates per serving

Note: If your digestive system is sensitive, either grind the nuts or omit.

Florentine-Stuffed Sole

YIELDS 4 SERVINGS

A healthy and delicious entrée with few calories.

1 package (10 ounces) frozen spinach, chopped
½ cup Easy Clarified Butter (page 37) or 100% pure, cold-pressed olive oil
1 teaspoon garlic powder
1 teaspoon each chopped fresh basil and oregano
½ teaspoon ground nutmeg
4 sole fillets (6 to 8 ounces each)
½ cup sliced or ground fresh raw almonds (see note)
1 medium lemon, scrubbed and sliced, for garnish
Fresh parsley sprigs for garnish

Preheat oven to 350°F. Thaw spinach in a microwave or colander; drain and squeeze out any liquid. Heat butter or oil in a large nonstick skillet; add spinach and seasonings. Mix well and remove from heat. Place spinach on the center of each fillet, reserving butter sauce in skillet. Roll fillets; secure with toothpicks. Place fillets into a greased 8-inch baking dish. Mix almonds into butter sauce; sprinkle over fillet tops. Bake 20 minutes; fillets are done when they flake at the touch of a fork. Garnish with lemon and parsley.

6 carbohydrates per serving

Note: If your digestive system is sensitive, either grind the nuts or omit.

Hearty Cioppino

YIELDS 4 SERVINGS

This bountiful and tasty cioppino is a winner!

*1 medium yellow onion,
scrubbed, peeled, and chopped*
*1 medium green bell pepper,
scrubbed and chopped*
*2 large cloves garlic, scrubbed,
peeled, and minced*
*4 large, fresh tomatoes,
scrubbed, peeled, cored, and
coarsely chopped*
*¼ cup 100% pure, cold-pressed
olive oil*
*2 tablespoons coarsely chopped
fresh parsley*

*1 tablespoon each coarsely
chopped fresh basil and thyme*
½ teaspoon sea salt (optional)
*1 dozen hard-shell clams,
scrubbed well*
*1 bass fillet (6 to 8 ounces), cut
into 2-inch chunks*
*1½ pounds fresh or frozen and
thawed crab (with shells,
scrubbed well)*
*¼ pound medium raw prawns,
peeled, deveined, and rinsed,
tails left on*

Place all ingredients, except bass, crab, and prawns, in a large
pot. Bring to a boil; reduce heat, cover, and simmer 30 minutes.
Add bass; simmer for 10 minutes. Add crab and prawns; cook 5
minutes longer, or until prawns turn pink. Serve hot.

5 carbohydrates per serving

Marinated Fish Kabobs

YIELDS 4 SERVINGS

The savory marinade is good on all grilled fish.

Fish Marinade

*½ cup 100% pure, cold-pressed
    olive oil*
2 tablespoons fresh lemon juice
*½ medium yellow onion, peeled,
    scrubbed, and chopped*

1 large clove garlic, minced
*1 tablespoon each chopped fresh
    oregano, thyme*
¼ teaspoon sea salt (optional)
Cayenne pepper to taste

Place all ingredients for marinade in a large dish or bowl.

*1½ pounds halibut, cut into
    2-inch squares*
*1 medium red bell pepper,
    scrubbed and cut into squares*

*1 medium yellow onion, peeled,
    scrubbed and cut into squares*

Add fish and red pepper and onion squares and marinate in refrigerator 2 hours or more, mixing occasionally. Before serving, alternate fish and vegetables on 4 large skewers. Place skewers on a broiling pan; broil. Or try barbecuing.

5 carbohydrates per serving of kabobs; 3 of marinade

Orange Roughy with Special Butter Sauce and Almonds

YIELDS 4 SERVINGS

Orange roughy is a white, low-fat fish from New Zealand—but sole may be used in its place. The special sauce creates a unique and delicious flavor and can be used with all types of fish and shellfish.

½ cup Easy Clarified Butter (page 00)
1 teaspoon each chopped fresh basil and oregano
Garlic powder to taste
4 orange roughy fillets (6 to 8 ounces each)

½ cup sliced or ground fresh almonds (see note)
1 medium lemon, scrubbed and cut into wedges, for garnish
Fresh parsley sprigs for garnish

Preheat oven to 350°F. Melt butter in a small skillet; add seasonings, mix and immediately remove from heat. Dip both sides of fish into butter sauce; place in a baking dish and pour any remaining sauce over tops of fillets. Sprinkle almonds over top. Bake 20 minutes. Test for doneness with a fork. Garnish with lemon and parsley.

3 carbohydrates per serving for sauce and almonds; 0 carbohydrates for fish

Note: If your digestive system is sensitive to sliced nuts, try grinding them instead, or omit.

Petrale Sole with Caviar and Butter Sauce

YIELDS 4 SERVINGS

This delicious and elegant recipe is extremely low in carbohydrates. Cooked baby shrimp may be used instead of caviar if you wish, and flounder is a good substitute for petrale sole.

4 ounces Easy Clarified Butter (page 37)
½ teaspoon garlic powder
1 teaspoon each chopped fresh basil and oregano
4 petrale sole fillets (6 to 8 ounces each)

1 jar (2.1 ounces) lumpfish caviar
½ medium red bell pepper, scrubbed and thinly sliced, for garnish
Fresh parsley sprigs for garnish

Preheat oven to 375°F. Melt butter in a small skillet. Add seasonings and herbs; mix and remove from heat. Place an 8-inch baking dish next to the skillet. Dip both sides of fillets in butter sauce; then place in baking dish, reserving butter in skillet. Bake 15 minutes, or until fork-tender. Place caviar in remaining butter sauce; mix gently. Spoon mixture over tops of fillets. Garnish with red bell pepper and parsley.

1 carbohydrate per serving

Sautéed Sole Monterey

YIELDS 2 SERVINGS

This flavorful recipe may be used for all kinds of fish.

2 large eggs
½ cup soy flour (see note)
¼ cup Easy Clarified Butter
(page 37) or 100% pure, cold-
pressed olive oil
2 tablespoons fresh lemon juice
2 tablespoons chopped fresh
parsley

½ teaspoon garlic powder
½ cup slivered or ground fresh
almonds
2 sole fillets (6 to 8 ounces each)
Fresh parsley sprigs for garnish
1 medium lemon, scrubbed and
sliced into thin rounds, for
garnish

Beat eggs in a small bowl; place flour in a shallow dish. Melt butter or oil in a large skillet; add lemon juice, parsley, garlic powder, and almonds; mix and remove from heat. Dip fillets into egg and then into flour; place in skillet. Sauté one side on medium-high heat until golden brown; turn. Brown other side. Garnish with parsley and lemon.

26 carbohydrates per serving

Note: If you're sensitive to soy, potato or rice flour may be used. If digestive system is sensitive, omit nuts or use ground nuts instead of slivered.

Seafood Extravaganza

YIELDS 2 SERVINGS

This is an impressive and delicious dish to serve someone special; it also has no carbohydrates.

¼ cup Easy Clarified Butter
(page 37) or 100% pure, cold-
pressed olive oil
½ teaspoon garlic powder
1 tablespoon each chopped fresh
basil and oregano
1 orange roughy or sole fillet (6
to 8 ounces)

¼ pound fresh or frozen and
thawed crab
¼ pound medium raw shrimp,
peeled, deveined, and rinsed,
tails left on
¼ pound sea or bay scallops

Preheat oven to 350°F. Melt butter in a large skillet; remove from heat. Add seasonings; mix. Place an 8-inch baking dish next to skillet. Cut orange roughy into 2-inch pieces. Dip into butter mixture and then place in a small baking dish, reserving butter mixture in skillet. Bake 10–15 minutes, or until fork-tender. Meanwhile, place crab, shrimp, and scallops into the remaining sauce in the skillet. Stir; turn for 3 minutes, or until shrimp is pink and scallops are cooked but not overdone. Remove orange roughy from oven; add to seafood skillet mixture. Mix gently; serve immediately.

0 carbohydrates per serving

Shrimp Amandine

YIELDS 4 SERVINGS

This tasty recipe may also be used for scallops or crab.

2 tablespoons Easy Clarified Butter (page 37) or 100% pure, cold-pressed olive oil
½ cup slivered or ground fresh almonds (see note)
1 medium red bell pepper, scrubbed and thinly sliced
1 cup cooked brown rice
1 can (17½ ounces) unsweetened chicken broth

1 package (10 ounces) frozen peas, thawed
¾ pound medium raw shrimp, peeled, deveined, and rinsed, tails left on
1 teaspoon garlic powder
½ teaspoon sea salt (optional)
1 tablespoon each chopped fresh dill, basil, and oregano

Melt butter or heat oil in a small skillet. Add almonds; sauté until lightly browned. Add bell pepper, rice, chicken broth, and peas. Mix; bring to a boil and reduce heat. Add shrimp, seasonings, and herbs; simmer just a few minutes, or until shrimp turns pink.

23 carbohydrates per serving

Note: If your digestive system is sensitive, remember that ground nuts are easier to digest than slivered or omit them altogether.

Shrimp and Rice Delight

YIELDS 6 SERVINGS

The combination of shrimp, snow peas, almonds, and bell pepper creates a gourmet casserole. Caution: This is high in carbohydrates.

1 cup raw brown rice
2¼ cups water (purified, preferably)
1 can (17½ ounces) unsweetened chicken broth
1 teaspoon sea salt (optional)
2 tablespoons 100% pure, cold-pressed olive oil
½ pound fresh snow peas, scrubbed

1 medium red bell pepper, scrubbed and thinly sliced
1 tablespoon each chopped fresh basil and oregano
½ cup sliced or ground fresh almonds (see note)
1 teaspoon garlic powder
¾ pound cooked baby shrimp, rinsed

Cook rice, water, broth, and salt in a 3-quart saucepan or electric frying pan, covered, for 1 hour, or until all liquid is absorbed. Heat oil in a large skillet; add vegetables, almonds, herbs, and seasonings; sauté until tender. Add shrimp; stir 2 minutes. Combine shrimp and rice mixtures in a large casserole; serve.

33 carbohydrates per serving

Note: If digestive system is sensitive, try ground instead of slivered almonds, or omit altogether.

Shrimp-Topped Rice Cakes

YIELDS 4 SERVINGS

Rice cakes are wonderful substitutions for bread and may also be topped with crab, salmon, tuna, chicken, or turkey.

*¼ pound cooked baby shrimp,
rinsed*
*1 stalk celery, scrubbed and
chopped*
*1 teaspoon each chopped fresh
dillweed and basil*
½ teaspoon garlic powder

*2 tablespoons Delicious Home-
made Mayonnaise (page 145)*
*1 large fresh tomato,
scrubbed and sliced into
four ¼-inch rounds*
4 rice cakes

Preheat oven to 350°F. Place shrimp, celery, seasonings, and mayonnaise in a small mixing bowl; blend. Place a tomato slice on each rice cake; place in a baking dish. Spoon shrimp mixture, divided equally, over tops of tomatoes. Cover with foil; bake 10 minutes, or until thoroughly heated.

10 carbohydrates per serving

Stuffed Half of Salmon

YIELDS 4 SERVINGS

This delicious stuffed salmon may be either baked or barbecued.

*¼ cup 100% pure, cold-pressed
olive oil*
*⅓ pound cooked baby shrimp,
rinsed and chopped*
*1 medium yellow onion,
scrubbed, peeled, and finely
chopped*
*1 medium lemon, with peel,
scrubbed and finely chopped*

*2 tablespoons finely chopped
fresh parsley*
*1 tablespoon chopped fresh
dillweed*
1 teaspoon garlic powder
½ teaspoon sea salt (optional)
*½ salmon (2–3 pounds), tail or
head left on*
Fresh parsley sprigs for garnish

Preheat oven to 350°F. Heat oil in a large skillet; add shrimp, onion, lemon, and seasonings. Sauté, mixing, for 1 minute; remove from heat and allow to cool. Stuff salmon with shrimp mixture; wrap in foil. Place in a baking dish; bake 45 minutes or barbecue 25–30 minutes. When fish flakes easily with a fork, it is done. Remove large bone before serving; garnish with parsley sprigs.

5 carbohydrates per serving

Stuffed Salmon for Two

YIELDS 2 SERVINGS

Because Stuffed Half of Salmon is so fabulous, this recipe was devised for just two people to enjoy.

*2 tablespoons Easy Clarified But-
ter (page 37) or 100% pure,
cold-pressed olive oil*
*¼ pound cooked baby shrimp,
rinsed and chopped*
*½ medium yellow onion,
scrubbed, peeled, and finely
chopped*
*½ medium lemon and peel,
scrubbed and finely chopped*

*1 tablespoon finely chopped fresh
parsley*
*½ tablespoon chopped fresh
dillweed*
½ teaspoon garlic powder
¼ teaspoon sea salt (optional)
*2 salmon fillets (6–8 ounces
each)*
Fresh parsley sprigs for garnish

Preheat oven to 350°F. Heat butter or oil in a small skillet; add shrimp, onion, lemon, and seasonings; mix and remove from heat. Cut fillets into halves. Place one half fillet (skin side down) in the center of a 12-inch piece of foil; repeat, using the other half fillet and placing on a second sheet of foil. Spread shrimp mixture over fillets on foil; top with other fillet halves (skin side up). Secure with toothpicks. Fold foil over fillets; seal. Place in an 8-inch baking dish; bake 25 minutes. Unwrap; test for doneness with a fork. Garnish with parsley sprigs.

6 carbohydrates per serving

Poultry

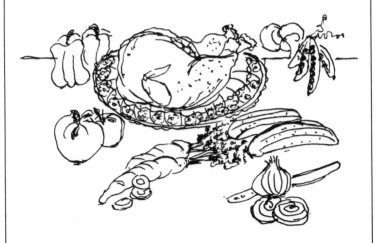

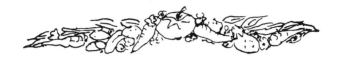

Chicken and Broccoli Delight

YIELDS 4 SERVINGS

This delicious dish may be served as a cold entrée.

1 frying chicken (approximately 3 pounds), quartered
2 medium new potatoes, scrubbed and peeled
½ pound fresh broccoli, scrubbed, trimmed, and sliced
½ cup Delicious Homemade Mayonnaise (page 145)
1 medium yellow onion, scrubbed, peeled, and chopped
2 tablespoons chopped fresh tarragon
1 teaspoon garlic powder
Sea salt to taste (optional)
½ cup chopped or ground fresh walnuts (see note)

Place chicken in a large kettle; cover with water. Heat to boiling uncovered; reduce heat and cover; simmer 45 minutes, or until fork-tender; cool. Remove skin and bones; cut into 1-inch cubes. Cook potatoes and broccoli separately until tender; drain, cool, and chop into 1-inch pieces. Mix chicken, potatoes, broccoli, mayonnaise, onion, and seasonings in a large bowl. Fold in nuts. This may be reheated in a microwave or oven before serving or served cold.

12 carbohydrates per serving

Note: If digestive system is sensitive, try ground nuts instead of chopped, or omit them altogether.

Chicken Cacciatore

YIELDS 4 SERVINGS

This wonderful chicken dish has very few carbohydrates, and any excess sauce is delicious served over brown rice.

1 frying chicken (approximately 3 pounds), quartered
1 teaspoon garlic powder, more or less, to taste
1 tablespoon chopped fresh oregano

1 tablespoon chopped fresh basil
1 can (8 ounces) unsweetened tomato sauce (without citric acid)

Preheat oven to 375°F. Place chicken quarters, skin side up, in a greased baking dish. Sprinkle seasonings over tops. Bake 30 minutes; turn and season with same spices. Bake 20 minutes longer. Spoon ½ can tomato sauce over chicken parts. Sprinkle more seasonings over sauce; turn and spoon rest of sauce over tops. Season and bake 10–15 minutes, or until tender.

2 carbohydrates per serving

Chicken Cutlets Italiano

YIELDS 4 SERVINGS

This is a very easy recipe to prepare and tasty as well.

¼ cup 100% pure, cold-pressed olive oil
2 eggs
⅓ cup brown rice flour
4 chicken cutlets (breast halves, skinned and boned)
1 cup scrubbed zucchini, sliced in ⅛-inch rounds

1 teaspoon garlic powder, more or less, to taste
1 tablespoon chopped fresh oregano
1 can (8 ounces) unsweetened tomato sauce (without citric acid)

Heat oil in a large nonstick skillet. Beat eggs in a small bowl. Spoon flour into a pie dish. Dip chicken breasts first into egg, next into flour, and then place in skillet; add zucchini. Sprinkle half of the seasonings over top; brown over medium-high heat. Turn; reduce heat. Spoon tomato sauce over cutlets and zucchini. Sprinkle remaining half of the seasonings over sauce. Simmer, covered, 10–15 minutes, or until fork-tender.

16 carbohydrates per serving

Chicken Thighs with Artichokes and Almonds

YIELDS 4 SERVINGS

Delicious marinated artichokes, rosemary, and almonds give chicken thighs fantastic flavor.

8 chicken thighs
Marinated Artichokes (page 122)
½ can (8¾ ounces) unsweetened
   chicken broth
2 tablespoons potato flour

1 teaspoon garlic powder, more
   or less, to taste
Sea salt to taste (optional)
Chopped fresh rosemary to taste
½ cup sliced almonds (see note)

Preheat oven to 350°F. Place chicken and artichokes in a greased 8-inch baking dish, reserving artichoke marinade. Bring broth to a boil in a 2-quart saucepan; reduce heat. Add marinade liquid, flour, and seasonings; mix until thick. Pour mixture over chicken and artichokes. Sprinkle more rosemary and almonds over top. Bake, uncovered, 30 minutes; baste with sauce. Cover; bake 20 minutes longer.

16 carbohydrates per serving

Note: If your digestive system is sensitive, try ground nuts or omit entirely.

Cornish Hens à L'Orange

YIELDS 4 SERVINGS

This is my favorite recipe for entertaining dinner guests because it has marvelous taste and elegant eye appeal. Wild Rice and Almonds (page 112) is a perfect accompaniment.

*1/4 cup Easy Clarified Butter
    (page 37) or 100% pure, cold-
    pressed olive oil
2 Rock Cornish hens, cut into
    halves
Garlic powder to taste*

*Chopped fresh tarragon to taste
1 1/2 cups unsweetened chicken
    broth
2 tablespoons potato flour
2 teaspoons special orange
    flavoring (see page 210)*

Preheat oven to 350°F. Heat butter or oil in a large skillet. Add hens. Sprinkle garlic powder and tarragon generously over tops. Brown one side on medium-high heat; turn, then season and brown the other side. Place in a 10-inch baking dish, reserving butter and seasonings in skillet. Add broth, flour, and orange flavoring to skillet mixture; stir just until well blended and smooth. Pour orange sauce over hens; cover and bake 1 hour, basting often. Serve any excess sauce with rice.

7 carbohydrates per serving

Florentine and Almond Chicken Rolls

YIELDS 4 SERVINGS

Scrumptious gourmet chicken rolls to satisfy any guest.

*1 package (10 ounces) frozen
    chopped spinach, thawed
4 chicken breast halves, skinned
    and boned
1/4 cup Easy Clarified Butter
    (page 37) or 100% pure, cold-
    pressed olive oil
1/2 teaspoon each chopped fresh
    basil and tarragon*

*Garlic powder and ground
    nutmeg to taste
1/2 cup sliced or ground fresh
    almonds (see note)
2 tablespoons melted Easy
    Clarified Butter*

Preheat oven to 350°F. Squeeze out any liquid from thawed spinach. Pound breasts to ⅛-inch thickness. Heat ¼ cup butter or oil in a small skillet. Add spinach and seasonings; mix and remove from heat. Spoon ¼ spinach mixture over top of each breast; roll and secure with toothpicks. Place breasts in an 8-inch baking dish. Heat almonds in butter; sprinkle over rolls. Bake 20 minutes, or until fork-tender, basting often. Cover when brown.

6 carbohydrates per serving

Note: Try ground nuts instead of sliced if your system is delicate.

Greek-Style Breast of Chicken

YIELDS 2–4 SERVINGS

This delicious, easy recipe, is courtesy of Tina Vasilious, of Belmont, California. When one isn't feeling up to doing much cooking, this is the perfect recipe because it takes little time to prepare and is tasty, nourishing, and very low in carbohydrates.

½ cup 100% pure, cold-pressed
  olive oil
Juice of 1 medium lemon,
  scrubbed before slicing

Chopped fresh oregano to taste
Garlic powder to taste
2–4 chicken breast halves,
  skinned (with bones)

Place a small bowl and foil-lined broiling pan next to each other. Place oil, lemon juice, and seasonings in bowl; mix. Dip both sides of chicken into the lemon–olive oil mixture and then place in broiling pan, reserving leftover sauce for basting. Broil one side until browned (about 5 minutes), basting often. Turn; broil other side, basting frequently until chicken is fork-tender.

2–3 carbohydrates per serving

Note: Several breasts can be broiled at one time, then frozen and reheated in the microwave or used in salads. They're also wonderful for bag lunches.

Lemon-Sautéed Chicken and Vegetables

YIELDS 2 SERVINGS

This is a delicious and easy-to-prepare dish. Brown rice is a perfect accompaniment to this entrée.

2 tablespoons 100% pure, cold-pressed olive oil
2 chicken breast halves, skinned and boned
1 medium lemon, scrubbed and cut in half
1 medium yellow onion, scrubbed, peeled, and sliced

1 scrubbed and coarsely shredded yellow crookneck squash
1 scrubbed and coarsely shredded zucchini
Garlic powder to taste
Chopped fresh tarragon to taste

Heat oil in a large skillet. Pound chicken to ⅛-inch thickness; place in skillet. Squeeze juice from ½ lemon over breasts; surround with onion, squash, and zucchini. Sprinkle seasoning over chicken and vegetables. Sauté over medium-high heat, stirring vegetables often. When one side is golden brown, turn; squeeze juice from other half of lemon over breasts and season again. Continue to sauté until chicken is golden brown, but not overdone.

13 carbohydrates per serving

Mexicali Chicken

YIELDS 3 SERVINGS

A delicious and unique way of coating chicken for a change. Spanish Brown Rice (page 110) is a perfect accompaniment.

1 package (9 ounces) tortilla chips
1 teaspoon garlic powder
Cayenne pepper to taste
½ cup Easy Clarified Butter (page 37), melted, or 100% pure, cold-pressed olive oil

1 frying chicken (approximately 3 pounds), cut into eighths

Preheat oven to 350°F. Crush tortilla chips in a food processor, or with a rolling pin on a board, into small flakes. Pour flakes into a shallow pan; add seasonings and mix. Pour melted butter or oil into a small bowl. Grease a 13 × 9-inch baking dish. Dip both sides of chicken first into butter or oil, next into flakes, then place in baking dish. Bake 30 minutes; turn and continue to bake 30 minutes longer.

18 carbohydrates per serving

Oriental Cashew Chicken

YIELDS 4 SERVINGS

This appealing dish depends on delicious bifun—Chinese wheat-free noodles.

2 tablespoons 100% pure, cold-pressed olive oil

2 chicken breast halves, skinned, boned, and cubed

2 stalks celery, without leaves, scrubbed and coarsely chopped

1 medium red bell pepper, scrubbed and thinly sliced

¼ pound fresh snow peas, scrubbed

3 small green onions, scrubbed, peeled, and chopped

1 clove garlic, scrubbed, peeled, and minced

½ cup whole or ground fresh cashew nuts (see note)

1 package (5 ounces) bifun, cooked and drained

1 tablespoon scrubbed and freshly grated gingerroot

½ teaspoon sea salt (optional)

1 tablespoon arrowroot powder

½ cup cold water (purified, preferably)

Heat oil in a large nonstick skillet. Add chicken, vegetables, and garlic; sauté until tender. Fold in cashews, noodles, and seasonings. Quickly mix arrowroot with water; add to mixture. Stir over medium heat until thick; serve.

28 carbohydrates per serving

Note: Ground cashews are easier to digest than whole or omit altogether.

Roasted Herb Chicken

YIELDS 4 SERVINGS

Chicken broth and wonderful fresh herbs make this a succulent dish. Brown rice is a good accompaniment.

1 whole roasting chicken (approximately 3 pounds)
100% pure, cold-pressed olive oil
Sea salt to taste (optional)

Chopped fresh rosemary and tarragon to taste
2 tablespoons potato flour
½ cup unsweetened chicken broth

Preheat oven to 350°F. Place chicken in a large baking dish or roasting pan. Rub oil over chicken; sprinkle seasonings over top and sides. Cover dish or pan with foil; bake 45 minutes, basting frequently. Remove foil; bake 15–20 minutes, or until browned. Remove from oven. Pour drippings into a 2-quart saucepan. Mix flour and broth in a measuring cup; pour into saucepan and stir until gravy thickens. Simmer 5 minutes. Cut chicken into serving pieces. Serve the gravy over the chicken, or on the side.

6 carbohydrates per serving

Special Baked Chicken and Zucchini

YIELDS 4 SERVINGS

This is a delicious way to serve chicken and zucchini.

*¼ cup 100% pure, cold-pressed
olive oil*
*1 frying chicken (approximately
3 pounds), quartered*
*1 large clove garlic, scrubbed,
peeled, and minced*
*Chopped fresh oregano and
thyme to taste (approximately
1 tablespoon each)*
*2 cups scrubbed and julienne-
shredded zucchini*

*1 tablespoon scrubbed and grated
fresh lemon peel*
*1 teaspoon garlic powder or to
taste*
*1 can (15 ounces) unsweetened
tomato sauce (without citric
acid)*
*1 tablespoon each fresh basil and
oregano*

Preheat oven to 375°F. Pour oil into a large skillet; add chicken
and garlic. Season with oregano and thyme; brown both sides of
chicken over medium-high heat. Cover; reduce heat and cook
30 minutes. Place chicken and zucchini in a greased, 13 × 9-inch
baking dish. Sprinkle lemon peel and garlic powder over top.
Cover with tomato sauce; season with basil and oregano. Cover
pan with foil; bake 30 minutes longer. Serve on a large platter.

11 carbohydrates per serving

Baked Lemon Turkey Breast

YIELDS 4 SERVINGS

This tasty turkey may be served either hot or chilled or used for salad.

½ fresh natural turkey breast (approximately 3–4 pounds)
½ can (8¾ ounces) unsweetened chicken broth (see note)
1 large clove garlic, scrubbed, peeled, and minced
1 medium lemon, scrubbed and sliced into rounds

1 medium yellow onion, scrubbed, peeled, and sliced
Chopped fresh sage and basil to taste
Sea salt to taste (optional)
Parsley sprigs for garnish

Preheat oven to 325°F. Place turkey in a large baking dish; cover with broth. Cut several slits in top of breast skin; plug with garlic. Place lemon slices on top of turkey; surround bottom of breast with onion. Sprinkle seasonings over breast; bake 20 minutes per pound, basting as needed. When browned, cover pan with foil; bake 30–50 minutes, or until fork-tender. Let sit a few minutes before slicing. Garnish with parsley before serving.

7 carbohydrates per serving

Note: to make gravy, add other half can of broth to residue in baking dish and use potato flour to thicken.

Turkey and Wild Rice Casserole

YIELDS 6 SERVINGS

Delicious chicken broth and other marvelous ingredients make a favorite dish. Caution: This is high in carbohydrates.

1 cup raw wild rice
¼ cup 100% pure, cold-pressed olive oil
1 medium yellow onion, scrubbed, peeled, and chopped
1 medium green bell pepper, scrubbed and diced
2 stalks celery, scrubbed and thinly sliced
¾ pound fresh natural turkey breast, cubed

8 ounces canned water chestnuts, drained and sliced
1 can (17½ ounces) unsweetened chicken broth
2 tablespoons potato or brown rice flour
1 teaspoon garlic powder
1 teaspoon chopped fresh sage

Preheat oven to 350°F. Rinse wild rice twice in colander under cold running water. Heat oil in an 8-inch nonstick skillet. Add onion, pepper, celery, and turkey; sauté until browned. Add water chestnuts, rice, and broth; mix. Add flour and seasonings; mix until well blended. Pour mixture into a 3-quart casserole. Cover; bake 45 minutes.

31 carbohydrates per serving

Meats

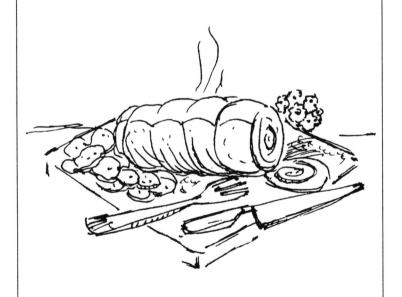

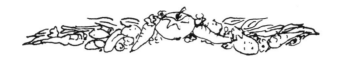

Beef and Broccoli Sauté

YIELDS 2 SERVINGS

This is a flavorful, quickly prepared entrée. Brown rice is a perfect accompaniment.

2 tablespoons 100% pure, cold-pressed olive oil
2 large cloves garlic, scrubbed, peeled, and minced
Grated scrubbed fresh gingerroot to taste
½ pound fresh broccoli, scrubbed, thinly sliced, and cut into 2-inch pieces

½ pound sirloin steak, thinly sliced and cut into 2-inch pieces (see note)
1 medium red bell pepper, scrubbed and thinly sliced
1 tablespoon arrowroot powder
¼ cup cold water (purified, preferably)

Heat oil in a large skillet; add garlic, ginger, broccoli, beef, and bell pepper. Sauté over medium-high heat, turning frequently, until meat is just browned. Mix arrowroot with water; add to skillet mixture. Stir until sauce thickens. Serve immediately.

15 carbohydrates per serving

Note: For a different taste, 2 chicken breasts, skinned and boned, may be used instead of beef.

Italian Pie with Zucchini Crust

YIELDS 6 SERVINGS

Zucchini makes a delicious pie crust for beef or chicken. Low in carbohydrates, too!

Zucchini Crust

2 cups scrubbed and coarsely
  grated zucchini
3 eggs, lightly beaten

2 tablespoons 100% pure, cold-
  pressed olive oil
1 teaspoon garlic powder

Preheat oven to 350°F. Mix all ingredients in a large bowl. Spoon mixture into a greased, 8-inch pie dish. Press against sides and bottom to form crust.

2 tablespoons 100% pure, cold-
  pressed olive oil
1 pound ground chuck, veal, or
  chicken
2 large cloves garlic, scrubbed,
  peeled, and minced

1 can (8 ounces) unsweetened
  tomato sauce (without citric
  acid)
½ teaspoon each chopped fresh
  oregano, sage, and basil

Heat oil in a large skillet; add meat and garlic. Brown, then drain off grease. Add tomato sauce and herbs; mix. Simmer, covered, for 10 minutes. Spoon into crust. Bake 30–40 minutes. 2 carbohydrates per serving for crust; 3 carbohydrates per serving for filling.

5 carbohydrates per serving

La Fiesta Mexicana

YIELDS 8 SERVINGS AS A MAIN DISH, MORE AS AN APPETIZER

This is a fabulous party dish that everyone will enjoy.

2 tablespoons 100% pure, cold-pressed olive oil
1 pound ground chuck steak, turkey, or chicken
Cayenne pepper and garlic powder to taste
Sea salt to taste (optional)
6 small green onions, scrubbed, peeled, and chopped
2 tablespoons 100% pure, cold-pressed olive oil

6 corn tortillas
2 cans (16 ounces each) vegetarian refried beans
1 head iceberg lettuce, scrubbed, dried, and shredded
8 cherry tomatoes, scrubbed and quartered
La Favorita Guacamole (page 45)
8 ounces tortilla chips

Preheat oven to 350°F. Heat oil in a large skillet. Sauté meat until browned; drain off grease. Add seasonings and green onions; mix and heat until tender; then remove from heat. Place tortillas into hot oil in another skillet; heat until bubbly on each side. Blot with paper towels; place in a large casserole. Spoon beans over tortillas; layer lettuce, meat mixture, and tomatoes over beans. Spread guacamole over layers. Top with chips. Cover with foil; bake 10–15 minutes.

25 carbohydrates per main-course serving

Marinated and Stuffed Flank Steak

YIELDS 4 SERVINGS

This plan-ahead entrée is very low in carbohydrates.

1½ pounds flank steak (have your butcher tenderize it)

Beef Marinade

*⅓ cup 100% pure, cold-pressed
   olive oil*
2 tablespoons fresh lemon juice
*1 medium yellow onion, scrubbed,
   peeled, and chopped*

*1 large clove garlic, scrubbed,
   peeled, and minced*

Place marinade ingredients in a small bowl; mix well and pour into a large baking dish. Place flank steak, unrolled, in marinade. Cover; refrigerate 2 hours to allow flavors to blend.

4 carbohydrates per serving of marinade.

Meat Stuffing

½ pound ground chuck or veal
1 large egg
*1 medium yellow onion,
   scrubbed, peeled, and finely
   chopped*

*2 tablespoons chopped fresh
   parsley*
Sea salt to taste (optional)

Preheat oven to 350°F. Mix stuffing ingredients; spread over flank steak. Roll flank steak lengthwise; secure with toothpicks. Bake, basting often, for 45 to 60 minutes, or until desired doneness.

4 carbohydrates per serving of stuffing

Meatballs with Sweet and Sour Sauce

YIELDS 4 SERVINGS AS A MAIN COURSE,
30 COCKTAIL-SIZE MEATBALLS AS AN APPETIZER

The impossible! Fabulous sweet and sour sauce! Brown rice or corn noodles are good accompaniments.

Meatballs

1 pound ground veal, turkey, or
  chicken
1 large egg
1 medium yellow onion,
  scrubbed, peeled, and finely
  grated

1 teaspoon chopped fresh basil
Curry powder to taste
1 teaspoon garlic powder

Mix all ingredients for meatballs in a large bowl; reserve for mixing with sauce. 4 carbohydrates per main-course serving.

16 carbohydrates per main-course serving

Sweet and Sour Sauce

1 can (8 ounces) unsweetened
  tomato sauce (without citric
  acid)
1 can (6 ounces) tomato paste
  (without citric acid)
1 tablespoon 100% pure, cold-
  pressed olive oil

1 teaspoon each, chopped fresh
  basil and oregano
1 teaspoon each, garlic powder
  and onion powder
5 tablespoons 100% Pure Vegetable Glycerine

Place all sauce ingredients in a large kettle; mix. Bring to a boil, then lower heat. Form balls with meat mixture; drop into sauce. Cover; simmer 1 hour.

16 carbohydrates per main-course serving

Mexican Spaghetti Pie

YIELDS 6 SERVINGS

Corn spaghetti makes this delicious pie crust. Caution: high in carbohydrates.

4 large eggs, beaten
Cayenne pepper to taste
½ teaspoon sea salt (optional)
½ package (6 ounces) corn
spaghetti, cooked and drained
2 tablespoons 100% pure, cold-
pressed olive oil
1 pound ground chuck, veal,
turkey, or chicken

1 medium yellow onion,
scrubbed, peeled, and chopped
1 large clove garlic, scrubbed,
peeled, and minced
2 large fresh tomatoes, scrubbed,
peeled, cored, puréed and
strained

Preheat oven to 375°F. Beat eggs in a large bowl. Add salt, cayenne pepper and spaghetti; gently mix with a wooden spoon. Pour mixture into a greased 9-inch pie plate; press against sides and bottom to form crust. Heat oil in a large skillet; sauté meat, onion, and garlic, turning frequently, until browned; drain off grease. Add tomatoes; mix and remove from heat. Pour mixture into crust. Place pie plate on a baking sheet; bake 30 minutes.

27 carbohydrates per serving

Curried Lamb Stew

YIELDS 4 SERVINGS

A perfect dish for entertaining on a cold night!

4 tablespoons 100% pure, cold-
pressed olive oil
1 pound lamb shoulder, cut into
bite-size pieces, fat trimmed
(see note)
¼ cup potato flour
1 medium yellow onion, scrubbed,
peeled, and chopped

2 medium new potatoes,
scrubbed, peeled, and diced
2 teaspoons curry powder
1 teaspoon garlic powder
½ teaspoon sea salt (optional)
1 package (10 ounces) frozen
peas, thawed

Preheat oven to 375°F. Heat oil in a large skillet. Coat lamb with flour. Add to oil, then add onion, potatoes, and seasonings. Sauté over medium-high heat until lightly browned, turning often. Add peas; stir mixture and remove from heat. Spoon into an 8-inch greased casserole. Bake 1 hour.

27 carbohydrates per serving

Note: 4 chicken breast halves, boned and skinned, may be substituted for the lamb.

Marinated Lamb Kabobs

YIELDS 4 SERVINGS

A special marinade gives lamb excellent flavor.

Marinade

2 large cloves garlic, scrubbed, peeled, and minced
1 medium yellow onion, scrubbed, peeled, and chopped
½ cup 100% pure, cold-pressed olive oil

¼ cup fresh lemon juice
1 teaspoon each chopped fresh oregano and thyme
1 teaspoon sea salt (optional)

Mix all marinade ingredients in a large bowl.

1½ pounds lamb, cut into 2-inch cubes, fat trimmed
2 medium green bell peppers, scrubbed and cut into 2-inch pieces

1 medium yellow onion, scrubbed, peeled, and cut into 2-inch pieces
8 cherry tomatoes, scrubbed

Place lamb and vegetables in marinade. Cover; refrigerate 3–4 hours; turn every hour. Alternate lamb and vegetables on skewers. Barbecue or broil each side 5 minutes or until browned.

12 carbohydrates per serving

Meat and Spinach Loaf

YIELDS 4 SERVINGS

This gourmet loaf combination has excellent flavor.

*1 package (10 ounces) frozen
    spinach, thawed, drained, and
    chopped
1 pound ground veal, chicken,
    or turkey
⅓ cup unsweetened soy milk (see
    note)
2 large eggs*

*1 medium yellow onion,
    scrubbed, peeled, and grated
Garlic powder and ground
    nutmeg to taste
2 medium new potatoes,
    scrubbed, peeled, and
    quartered
Ground paprika to taste*

Preheat oven to 350°F. Place spinach, meat, milk, eggs, onion, and seasonings in a large bowl; mix. Form a loaf; place in a greased 8-inch baking dish. Spread topping (below) over loaf. Surround loaf with potatoes, season with paprika. Bake 45–55 minutes.

25 carbohydrates per serving with topping; 20 carbohydrates without

Tomato Topping

*6 tablespoons tomato paste (with-
    out citric acid)
¼ cup fresh lemon juice*

*Chopped fresh oregano and
    basil to taste*

Mix all ingredients in a small bowl; spread over meat loaf.

5 carbohydrates per serving for 4

Note: If you're sensitive to soy, use nut milk or egg whites instead (see "Dairy Substitutes").

Meatballs and Spaghetti

YIELDS 4 SERVINGS

Soba, pure buckwheat spaghetti, is delicious with these meatballs. Caution: This is high in carbohydrates.

1 pound ground veal, turkey, or chicken
1 medium yellow onion, scrubbed, peeled, and finely grated
2 tablespoons coarsely chopped fresh parsley

1 teaspoon garlic powder
1 tablespoon coarsely chopped fresh oregano
1 large egg

Mix all ingredients in a large bowl; drop into sauce below.

4 carbohydrates per serving

Special Spaghetti Sauce

YIELDS 4 SERVINGS

1 can (15 ounces) unsweetened tomato sauce (without citric acid)
1 can (6 ounces) tomato paste (without citric acid)
2 tablespoons coarsely chopped fresh parsley
2 tablespoons 100% pure, cold-pressed olive oil

1 tablespoon each coarsely chopped fresh basil and oregano

1 package (7 ounces) cooked and drained soba noodles

Place sauce ingredients in a large kettle; heat. Bring to a boil; cover and simmer 1 hour. Serve over soba noodles.

16 carbohydrates per serving for 4 without soba; add 21 for soba

Veal Paupiettes with Gourmet Sauce

YIELDS 4 SERVINGS

This is a delicious and impressive way of entertaining dinner guests.

½ pound ground veal
1 large egg
½ medium yellow onion,
*   scrubbed, peeled, and chopped*
1 teaspoon chopped fresh
*   tarragon*

¼ teaspoon sea salt (optional)
4 large veal steak slices, pounded
*   thin*

Place ground veal, egg, onion, tarragon, and salt in a large bowl; mix. Spread ¼ mixture over top of each steak slice; roll and secure with toothpicks. Cover; reserve for Gourmet Sauce (below).

2 carbohydrates per serving

Gourmet Sauce

3 tablespoons 100% pure, cold-
*   pressed olive oil*
2 green onions, scrubbed, peeled,
*   and finely chopped*

1 large clove garlic, scrubbed,
*   peeled, and minced*
½ teaspoon fresh rosemary,
*   chopped*

Heat oil in a large skillet. Add onions, garlic, and rosemary; mix. Add meat rolls to skillet. Lightly brown each side 3 minutes over medium-high heat. Cover; simmer 10 minutes or until thoroughly cooked.

3 carbohydrates per serving

Pastas,
Rice, and
Other Grains

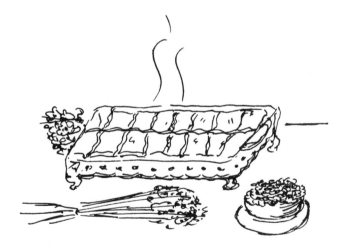

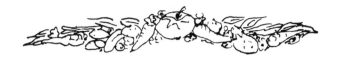

Delicious Lokchen Kugel
(Noodle Pudding)

YIELDS 6 SERVINGS

This delicious dish, of Eastern European origin, is made with corn noodles.

2 large eggs
1 cup raw cottage cheese (see note)
1/4 cup Easy Clarified Butter (page 37)
1 tablespoon scrubbed and grated fresh lemon peel
2 tablespoons 100% Pure Vegetable Glycerine

1 teaspoon special vanilla flavoring (see page 210)
2 teaspoons ground cinnamon, divided
1/2 pound corn ribbons (noodles), cooked and drained
Easy Clarified Butter

Mock Sour Cream (page 40)

Preheat oven to 350°F. Beat eggs in a large bowl until light. Add cottage cheese, butter, lemon peel, glycerine, vanilla, and 1 teaspoon cinnamon; mix well. Fold in noodles. Pour mixture into a greased 8-inch baking dish. Sprinkle 2 tablespoons butter and 1 teaspoon cinnamon over top. Bake 45 minutes, or until brown. Serve warm with Mock Sour Cream.

33 carbohydrates per serving

Note: If digestive system is sensitive, do not use raw cottage cheese, try plain low-fat yogurt instead.

107

Linguini with Clams and Garlic Sauce

YIELDS 4 SERVINGS

Soba, a Japanese wheat-free spaghetti, makes a delicious substitute for wheat-based linguini with this recipe.

¼ cup Easy Clarified Butter (page 37) or 100% pure, cold-pressed olive oil
2 large cloves garlic, scrubbed, peeled, and minced
1 can (6½ ounces) unsweetened minced clams (without MSG), drained

1 tablespoon chopped fresh parsley
1 package (7 ounces) soba (100% pure buckwheat spaghetti)

Melt butter in a large skillet. Add garlic; sauté until tender. Add clams and parsley; simmer. Prepare soba noodles while the sauce is cooking, then drain. Immediately serve sauce mixed into or poured over soba.

22 carbohydrates per serving

Deep-Fried Croquettes

YIELDS 16 CROQUETTES

Quinoa is a wonderful grain, full of protein.

2 cups cooked quinoa
2 large green onions, scrubbed, peeled, and finely chopped
2 tablespoons finely chopped fresh parsley
1 teaspoon each chopped fresh marjoram and basil
½ teaspoon chopped fresh sage

½ teaspoon sea salt (optional)
2 tablespoons, more or less, brown rice flour
2 tablespoons, more or less, water (purified, preferably)
2 cups 100% pure, cold-pressed olive oil

Place quinoa, green onions, herbs, and salt in a large bowl; mix. Add just enough flour and water so that mixture sticks together. Form 16 balls. Place oil in a large skillet or wok; heat to 375°F. Gently drop each ball into skillet; cook 4 minutes, or until croquettes are golden brown. Remove from heat; drain on paper towels. Serve immediately or keep warm in oven.

4 carbohydrates each

Mock Tabooli

YIELDS 4 SERVINGS

Quinoa substitutes for the wheat in tabooli.

½ cup raw quinoa
1 cup water (purified, preferably)
2 tablespoons chopped fresh parsley
6 small green onions, scrubbed, peeled, and chopped
1 large clove garlic, scrubbed, peeled, and minced
½ cup 100% pure, cold-pressed olive oil

½ cup fresh lemon juice
2 tablespoons chopped fresh mint
1 tablespoon chopped fresh basil
Sea salt to taste (optional)
1 can (2.2 ounces) sliced ripe olives, drained (optional)
4 large lettuce leaves, scrubbed and dried

Rinse quinoa; drain. Combine with water in a 2-quart saucepan; bring to a boil. Reduce heat; simmer, uncovered, 10 minutes, or until all liquid is absorbed. Mix all ingredients, except lettuce, in a large bowl. Refrigerate mixture 1–2 hours. Serve over lettuce.

22 carbohydrates per serving

Spanish Brown Rice

YIELDS 4 SERVINGS

Brown rice makes delicious Spanish rice; it's a perfect accompaniment to Mexicali Chicken (page 86). Caution: This is high in carbohydrates.

1 cup water (purified, preferably)
½ cup raw brown rice
¼ teaspoon sea salt (optional)
2 tablespoons 100% pure, cold-pressed olive oil
1 medium yellow onion, scrubbed, peeled, and chopped

1 medium green bell pepper, scrubbed and chopped
½ cup chopped fresh parsley
2 large fresh tomatoes, scrubbed, peeled, cored, and coarsely chopped
Cayenne pepper to taste

Bring water to a boil in a 1-quart saucepan. Add rice and salt. Reduce heat, cover, and simmer 40 minutes, or until all liquid is absorbed. Heat oil in a large nonstick skillet. Add rice and rest of ingredients. Sauté over medium-high heat, stirring frequently until vegetables are tender.

26 carbohydrates per serving

Special Lemon Rice

YIELDS 4 SERVINGS

This delicious and unique rice dish is a wonderful accompaniment to fish, shellfish, and chicken entrées.

1⅓ cups water (purified, preferably)
½ cup raw brown rice
½ teaspoon sea salt (optional)
2 tablespoons 100% pure, cold-pressed olive oil
½ medium yellow onion, scrubbed, peeled, and finely chopped

1 tablespoon finely chopped fresh parsley
½ medium lemon, scrubbed and chopped
1 teaspoon garlic powder

Bring water to a boil. Add rice and salt. Reduce heat; cover and simmer 15–20 minutes, or until all liquid is absorbed. Heat oil in a large nonstick skillet; sauté onion and parsley until tender. Add cooked rice, lemon, and garlic powder. Mix well; cover and simmer 5–10 minutes.

22 carbohydrates per serving

Wild Rice and Almonds

YIELDS 6 SERVINGS

This elegant rice dish is a perfect accompaniment to turkey, chicken, or Cornish hen entrées.

1 cup raw wild rice
Water (purified, preferably)
1 teaspoon sea salt (optional)
2 tablespoons 100% pure, cold-pressed olive oil
1 large clove garlic, scrubbed, peeled, and minced
2 stalks celery, without leaves, scrubbed and coarsely chopped

1 medium yellow onion, scrubbed, peeled, and coarsely chopped
½ cup chopped fresh parsley
½ cup slivered or ground fresh almonds (see note)

Boil wild rice with 2 cups water for 1 minute; drain. Repeat process. Then place rice, 3 cups water, and salt in a 3-quart saucepan. Cover and simmer 35 minutes, or until kernels puff open; drain. Pour oil into a large skillet, sauté garlic, celery, onion, and parsley until tender. Add almonds and cooked rice; mix well. Simmer, covered, 15 minutes, or place rice mixture into a greased mold and bake in a preheated 350°F oven for 20–30 minutes. Serve hot with entrée.

25 carbohydrates per serving

Note: Try ground almonds rather than slivered for an easier-to-digest dish.

Wild Rice Pudding

YIELDS 4 SERVINGS

This pudding is a delicious and welcome change. Caution: This is high in carbohydrates.

2 large eggs
2 tablespoons 100% Pure Vegetable Glycerine
1 teaspoon vanilla flavoring
½ teaspoon ground cinnamon
¼ teaspoon ground nutmeg

¼ teaspoon sea salt (optional)
½ cup raw wild rice, cooked
1 cup unsweetened soy milk (see note)
Ground cinnamon for garnish

Preheat oven to 350°F. Beat eggs in a large bowl. Mix in rest of the ingredients, except cinnamon, for garnish. Pour into greased 6 individual custard cups. Sprinkle cinnamon over tops. Place cups in a baking pan with water. Bake 1 hour, or until firm. Serve warm or cold.

32 carbohydrates per serving

Note: If your system is sensitive to soy, try nut milk or egg whites instead (see "Dairy Substitutes").

Wild Rice Stuffing

YIELDS 4 SERVINGS

This wild rice recipe is a wonderful substitution for traditional bread stuffing for chicken, Cornish hens, and turkey. Caution: It's high in carbohydrates.

1 cup raw wild rice
¼ cup Easy Clarified Butter
(page 37)
½ cup chopped or ground fresh almonds (see note)
2 stalks celery, scrubbed and chopped

1 medium yellow onion, scrubbed, peeled, and chopped
1 can (17½ ounces) unsweetened chicken broth
1 teaspoon garlic powder
1 tablespoon chopped fresh sage
Sea salt to taste (optional)

Rinse wild rice twice in colander under cold water. Heat butter in a large nonstick skillet. Add almonds, celery, and onion; sauté until tender. Mix in broth, seasonings, and rice. If stuffing a turkey bake in a preheated 325°F oven for 20 minutes per pound; or place stuffing in a greased 2-quart baking dish or casserole and bake, covered, in preheated 350°F oven 45–55 minutes.

40 carbohydrates per serving

Note: Ground nuts are easier to digest than chopped.

Yakimeshi (Japanese Fried Rice)

YIELDS 4 SERVINGS

A mixture of shrimp, snow peas, and other flavorful ingredients create this sensational dish.

2 tablespoons 100% pure, cold-pressed olive oil
½ cup raw brown rice, cooked
¼ pound fresh snow peas, scrubbed
3 small green onions, scrubbed, peeled, and chopped

Grated, scrubbed fresh gingerroot to taste
½ teaspoon garlic powder
3 large eggs
½ pound cooked baby shrimp, rinsed (optional)

Heat oil in a large nonstick skillet or wok. Add cooked rice, snow peas, green onions, and seasonings. Sauté, over medium-high heat, for a few minutes, mixing and turning. Reduce heat to medium. Make a well in center of rice mixture. Drop unbeaten eggs into well; stir. Add shrimp; stir 2 minutes or until eggs are set. Serve immediately.

23 carbohydrates per serving

Vegetables

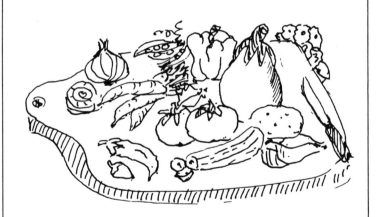

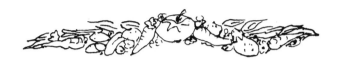

Asparagus Sauté

YIELDS 4 SERVINGS

Fresh ginger, garlic, and sesame seeds give asparagus delicious flavor.

*1 pound fresh asparagus,
scrubbed and cut on the
diagonal into 2-inch pieces*
Water (purified, preferably)
*2 tablespoons 100% pure, cold-
pressed olive oil*

*Grated scrubbed fresh gingerroot
to taste*
*2 large cloves garlic, scrubbed,
peeled, and minced*
½ teaspoon sea salt (optional)
2 tablespoons sesame seeds

Place asparagus in a large pot; cover with water. Bring to a boil, reduce heat, and cook 5 minutes; drain. Heat oil in a large skillet. Add ginger, garlic, salt, sesame seeds, and asparagus. Sauté, stirring and turning frequently, until tender.

5 carbohydrates per serving

Broccoli and Easy Hollandaise Sauce

YIELDS 4 SERVINGS

What a delicious way to serve broccoli—and so low in carbohydrates, too!

2 tablespoons 100% pure, cold-pressed olive oil
2 large cloves garlic, scrubbed, peeled, and minced
1 pound fresh broccoli, scrubbed and cut into spears

1 teaspoon each coarsely chopped fresh tarragon and basil

Easy Hollandaise Sauce (page 177)

Pour oil into a large nonstick skillet. Add garlic; sauté 2 minutes or until tender. Place broccoli and seasonings in skillet; sauté over medium-high heat 5–10 minutes, turning frequently, until fork-tender. Serve Easy Hollandaise Sauce either over broccoli or separately.

5 carbohydrates per serving

Cabbage Sauté

YIELDS 4 SERVINGS

This is a delicious way to prepare cabbage. Potato flour is a wonderful thickener, and caraway adds perfect flavor.

¼ cup, or more, Easy Clarified Butter (page 37)
1 green cabbage (approximately 1 pound), scrubbed and shredded
1 medium yellow onion, scrubbed, peeled, and thinly sliced

2 tablespoons potato flour
1 tablespoon caraway seeds
Sea salt to taste (optional)

Melt butter in a large, nonstick skillet. Add cabbage and onion. Sauté over medium-high heat 5 minutes, stirring often. Lower heat. Add flour; mix. Add more butter, if needed, then add caraway seeds and salt. Mix and continue to cook over low heat 5 minutes, or until tender.

13 carbohydrates per serving

Eggplant Supreme

YIELDS 2 SERVINGS

This scrumptious recipe may be used as a main dish, with or without meat.

1 eggplant (approximately 1 pound), scrubbed
2 large eggs
2 tablespoons 100% pure, cold-pressed olive oil
½ pound ground chuck, veal, or chicken (optional)

1 can (8 ounces) unsweetened tomato sauce (without citric acid)
1 tablespoon each coarsely chopped fresh basil and oregano

Preheat oven to 350°F. Cut eggplant in half. Scoop out edible fruit; reserve shells. Cut fruit into 1-inch chunks. Beat eggs in a large bowl. Place eggplant chunks into beaten eggs; soak 5 minutes. Meanwhile, heat oil in a large nonstick skillet. Add meat; sauté until browned; drain off grease. Add eggplant chunks; sauté, turning often, until golden brown. Add tomato sauce and seasonings. Place shells in an 8-inch baking dish, filling them with skillet mixture. Bake, uncovered, for 45 minutes, or until shells are tender.

18 carbohydrates per serving

Florentine-Stuffed Tomatoes

YIELDS 4 SERVINGS

This is a delicious luncheon recipe and looks elegant too!

1 package (10 ounces) frozen chopped spinach, thawed and drained
4 large fresh tomatoes, scrubbed
2 tablespoons 100% pure, cold-pressed olive oil
1 large clove garlic, scrubbed, peeled, and minced

1 medium yellow onion, scrubbed, peeled, and finely chopped
1 tablespoon coarsely chopped fresh basil
½ teaspoon ground nutmeg
¼ cup ground fresh almonds

Preheat oven to 400°F. Squeeze out all liquid from spinach. Cut tops off tomatoes; remove pulp. Chop pulp; place into a small bowl and reserve. Heat oil in a large skillet. Add garlic and onion; sauté until tender. Add spinach, tomato pulp, basil and nutmeg. Stir; turn until spinach and tomato are well coated with seasonings; remove from heat. Place tomatoes in a buttered, 8-inch baking dish; fill with spinach mixture. Top with almonds. Bake 15–20 minutes.

14 carbohydrates per serving

Marinated Artichokes

YIELDS 8 ARTICHOKE HALVES

Marinated artichokes are delicious as appetizers or in salads. I also use them in Baked Chicken Thighs with Artichokes and Almonds (page 83).

4 fresh Jerusalem or miniature artichokes, scrubbed and trimmed

Water (purified, preferably)
Italian Dressing and Marinade (page 146)

Place artichokes in a 2-quart saucepan. Add enough water to cover tops; bring to a boil. Cover; cook over medium heat 10–15 minutes, or until leaves are very tender. Remove from heat; drain and cool. Pull off any tough outer leaves; slice artichokes in half. Place in Italian Dressing and Marinade. If marinade does not completely cover artichokes, add a little more cold water. Refrigerate overnight or for several hours to allow flavors to blend.

24 carbohydrates; 3 per artichoke half

Scrumptious Zucchini Sauté

YIELDS 4 SERVINGS

A delicious easy, low-carbohydrate way to prepare zucchini!

2 tablespoons 100% pure, cold-pressed olive oil

2 large cloves garlic, scrubbed, peeled, and minced

1 pound zucchini, scrubbed and julienne-shredded or cut into thin matchsticks

1 large tomato, scrubbed and coarsely chopped

3 small green onions, scrubbed, peeled, and coarsely chopped

Coarsely chopped fresh basil to taste

Sea salt to taste (optional)

Heat oil in a large nonstick skillet. Add garlic; sauté 2–3 minutes until tender. Add rest of ingredients; sauté, turning frequently, 2–3 minutes until cooked but not overdone.

7 carbohydrates per serving

South-of-the-Border Beans

YIELDS 8 SERVINGS

This is a very hearty and flavorful bean recipe. Caution: It's high in carbohdyrates.

1 pound dried black beans, washed thoroughly, soaked overnight, and drained
Water (purified, preferably)
¼ cup 100% pure, cold-pressed olive oil
2 medium yellow onions, scrubbed, peeled, and coarsely chopped

1 medium green bell pepper, scrubbed and coarsely chopped
4 stalks celery, without leaves, scrubbed and chopped
4 large cloves garlic, scrubbed, peeled, and minced
1 teaspoon sea salt (optional)
⅛ teaspoon ground cumin
Cayenne pepper to taste

Place beans in a large kettle; cover with water. Bring to a boil; lower heat and simmer 2 minutes; drain. Repeat process twice more; remove from heat. Heat oil in a large skillet. Add vegetables and seasonings; sauté until tender. Add to pot of beans; mix. Cover; cook 2 hours, adding a little more water if mixture is too thick.

36 carbohydrates per serving

Savory Lima Beans

YIELDS 6 SERVINGS

Garbanzo flour highlights this tasty recipe.

1 pound dried lima beans, washed thoroughly, soaked overnight, and drained

Water (purified, preferably)

2 tablespoons 100% pure, cold-pressed olive oil

1 medium yellow onion, scrubbed, peeled, and coarsely chopped

1 large clove garlic, scrubbed, peeled, and minced

2 tablespoons garbanzo flour

Cayenne pepper to taste

1 teaspoon sea salt (optional)

1 can (8 ounces) unsweetened tomato sauce (without citric acid)

1 can (6 ounces) tomato paste (without citric acid)

1 tablespoon 100% Pure Vegetable Glycerine

Preheat oven to 350°F. Place beans in a large kettle; cover with water. Bring to a boil; lower heat and simmer 2 minutes; drain. Repeat process twice more. Add water to cover beans; simmer, covered, 30 minutes. Sauté onion and garlic in oil until tender. Place garlic, onion, beans and liquid, and rest of ingredients in an 8-inch casserole; mix. Bake 45 minutes, or until tender.

23 carbohydrates per serving

Spinach Soufflé

YIELDS 4 SERVINGS

This elegant soufflé is a delicious accompaniment to meat, fish, and poultry entrées.

¼ cup Easy Clarified Butter (page 37) or 100% pure, cold-pressed olive oil
1 medium white onion, scrubbed, peeled, and finely chopped
1 package (10 ounces) frozen chopped spinach, thawed and drained

4 large eggs, beaten
1 teaspoon ground nutmeg
¼ teaspoons sea salt (optional)
2 ounces sliced or ground fresh almonds (see note)

Preheat oven to 350°F. Melt butter in a large skillet. Add onion; stir and sauté over medium-high heat until tender. Add spinach, onion, and seasonings to beaten eggs; mix and pour into a greased 2-quart baking dish. Bake 30 minutes, or until firm. Top with almonds.

9 carbohydrates per serving

Note: Remember: Ground almonds are easier to digest than sliced, or omit altogether.

Spinach Quiche

YIELDS 6 SERVINGS

The delicious pecan crust and flavorful spinach/cheese filling make this dish a gourmet delight.

1 package (10 ounces) frozen chopped spinach, thawed and drained
¼ cup Easy Clarified Butter (page 37) or 100% pure, cold-pressed olive oil
1 medium yellow onion, scrubbed, peeled, and finely chopped

4 large eggs
¾ cup raw cottage cheese (see note)
½ teaspoon ground nutmeg
½ teaspoon chopped fresh basil
¼ teaspoon sea salt (optional)
Perfect Pecan Crust (page 193)

Preheat oven to 325°F. Squeeze out any liquid from spinach. Heat butter or oil in a small nonstick skillet; sauté onion until tender. Beat eggs in a large bowl. Mix spinach and onion into egg. Add cottage cheese and seasonings; mix well. Spoon into Perfect Pecan Crust. Bake 30 minutes, or until firm.

8 carbohydrates per serving

Note: If digestive system is sensitive, do not try raw cottage cheese; try fresh drained tofu, if tolerated.

Sweet Yam Casserole

YIELDS 4 SERVINGS

Glycerine and orange flavoring combine to make this recipe a sweet success!

1/4 cup water (purified, preferably)
2 tablespoons 100% Pure Vege-
table Glycerine
2 teaspoons special orange
flavoring (see page 210)

Ground cinnamon to taste
1/2 cup chopped or ground
fresh walnuts (see note)
1/2 pound yams, scrubbed,
peeled, and quartered

Preheat oven to 350°F. Place yams in a greased 8-inch casserole. Put all other ingredients into a small bowl; mix. Pour mixure over yams and bake 35 minutes, or until fork-tender.

14 carbohydrates per serving

Note: Try ground nuts if your system is sensitive, or omit altogether.

Gourmet Zucchini Casserole

YIELDS 4 SERVINGS

This scrumptious, colorful, easy-to-prepare casserole is a fine accompaniment to any entrée.

*2 cups scrubbed and thinly sliced
green zucchini rounds*
*1 cup scrubbed and thinly sliced
golden zucchini rounds*
*1 medium red bell pepper,
scrubbed and thinly sliced*

*2 tablespoons 100% pure, cold-
pressed olive oil*
*1 teaspoon garlic powder, or
more, to taste*
*Coarsely chopped fresh basil and
oregano to taste*

Preheat oven to 375°F. Place green zucchini, golden zucchini, and bell pepper slices alternately into a greased 8-inch casserole. Mix oil and seasonings; sprinkle over vegetables. Bake 20–30 minutes.

5 carbohydrates per serving

Zucchini-Tomato Melt

YIELDS 4 SERVINGS

Rice cakes are wonderful substitutes for bread and make delicious hot open-faced sandwiches in this recipe.

*2 tablespoons 100% pure, cold-
pressed olive oil*
*1 cup scrubbed and thinly sliced
zucchini rounds*
*1 large fresh tomato, scrubbed
well and coarsely chopped*

*1 medium yellow onion,
scrubbed and chopped fine*
Garlic powder to taste
Chopped fresh basil to taste
4 rice cakes

Preheat oven to 350°F. Heat oil in a large skillet. Add zucchini, tomato, onion, and seasonings; sauté until tender. Remove from heat. Place rice cakes in a baking dish. Spoon skillet mixture onto cakes; cover dish with foil. Bake 10 minutes, or until thoroughly heated.

14 carbohydrates per serving

Salads
and
Salad Dressings

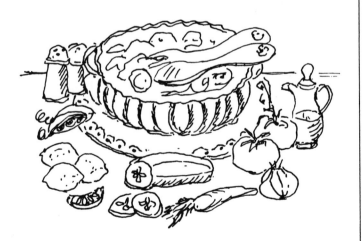

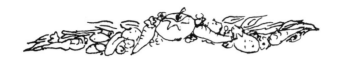

Cantonese Chicken Salad

YIELDS 4 SERVINGS

This delicious salad is very low in carbohydrates.

5 tablespoons cold-pressed
   sesame oil
2 cups water (purified,
   preferably)
3 chicken breast halves
2 cups scrubbed and shredded
   iceberg lettuce
2 cups scrubbed and shredded
   red cabbage

3 small green onions, scrubbed,
   peeled, and finely chopped
2 tablespoons 100% Pure Vegetable Glycerine
Grated scrubbed fresh gingerroot
   to taste
2 tablespoons coarsely chopped
   fresh parsley
2 tablespoons sesame seeds

Heat 1 tablespoon of the sesame oil with the water in a 3-quart saucepan. Add chicken; simmer, covered, for 15 minutes, or until tender. Remove chicken from pot; cool. Skin and bone chicken; shred into a large bowl. Add remaining sesame oil and rest of ingredients; mix. Cover and refrigerate 1–2 hours before serving.

5 carbohydrates per serving

Curried Turkey and Almond Salad

YIELDS 4 SERVINGS

The wonderful blend of curry and Delicious Homemade Mayonnaise makes a delightful salad.

½ pound cooked natural turkey breast, cubed

2 large eggs, hard-cooked, peeled, and coarsely chopped

2 stalks celery, without leaves, scrubbed and coarsely chopped

3 small green onions, scrubbed, peeled, and coarsely chopped

1 medium red bell pepper, scrubbed and coarsely chopped

¼ cup Delicious Homemade Mayonnaise (page 145)

Curry powder to taste

4 large lettuce leaves, scrubbed and dried

¼ cup slivered or ground fresh almonds (see note)

Place all ingredients, except lettuce and almonds, in a large bowl; mix well. Place lettuce leaves on 4 salad plates. Spoon salad over leaves. Sprinkle almonds over tops.

5 carbohydrates per serving

Note: If your digestive system is sensitive, remember: Ground nuts are easier to digest than slivered. Or omit the nuts altogether.

Delicious Shrimp Louis

YIELDS 4 SERVINGS

Fresh herbs, Delicious Homemade Mayonnaise, and other tasty ingredients make this a favorite salad.

½ pound cooked baby shrimp, rinsed (see note)
2 large eggs, hard-cooked, peeled, and grated
1 medium cucumber, scrubbed, peeled, and diced
3 small green onions, scrubbed, peeled, and finely chopped
2 stalks celery, without leaves, scrubbed and coarsely chopped
1 tablespoon coarsely chopped fresh parsley

2 tablespoons coarsley chopped fresh basil
¼ cup Delicious Homemade Mayonnaise (page 145)
4 romaine lettuce leaves, scrubbed and dried
8 fresh asparagus spears, scrubbed, trimmed, cooked, and cooled

Mix all ingredients, except romaine and asparagus, in a large bowl. Place romaine on 4 salad plates. Spoon salad, equally divided, onto each romaine leaf; garnish with whole asparagus spears. Chill before serving.

5 carbohydrates per serving

Note: Crab, tuna, chicken, or turkey may be used instead of shrimp.

Fancy Red and Green Slaw

YIELDS 4 SERVINGS

The delightful flavor of this salad comes from Delicious Home-made Mayonnaise, Glycerine, and caraway seeds.

1 green cabbage (approximately 1 pound), scrubbed and grated
1 red cabbage (approximately 1 pound), scrubbed and grated
3 green onions, scrubbed, peeled, and finely chopped
¼ cup Delicious Homemade Mayonnaise (page 145)

1 tablespoon 100% Pure Vegetable Glycerine
2 teaspoons caraway seeds (see note)
Sea salt to taste

Mix all ingredients in a large bowl. Refrigerate at least 1 hour before serving to allow flavors to blend.

7 carbohydrates per serving

Note: If digestive system is sensitive, omit caraway seeds.

Favorite Potato Salad

YIELDS 4–6 SERVINGS

This colorful and delicious potato salad is perfect for any occasion, from a casual picnic to a party buffet.

4 medium new potatoes, scrubbed, peeled, and cooked (in purified water, preferably)
2 eggs, hard-cooked, peeled, and coarsely chopped
1 medium cucumber, scrubbed, peeled, and diced
2 stalks celery, without leaves, scrubbed and coarsely chopped
3 small green onions, scrubbed, peeled, and coarsely chopped

5 medium radishes, scrubbed and diced
¼ cup Delicious Homemade Mayonnaise (page 145)
3 tablespoons chopped fresh parsley
1 teaspoon celery salt
½ teaspoon dry mustard
1 can (2.2 ounces) chopped olives, drained (optional)

Cook potatoes in enough water to cover, cool. Dice potatoes and place in a large bowl. Add rest of ingredients, except olives; mix. Gently fold in olives. Refrigerate at least 1–2 hours before serving.

20 carbohydrates per serving for 4; 14 carbohydrates per serving for 6

Gourmet Tuna-Stuffed Tomatoes

YIELDS 2 SERVINGS

Delicious Homemade Mayonnaise, fresh herbs, and almonds enhance standard tuna salad.

2 large lettuce leaves, scrubbed and dried
2 large fresh tomatoes, scrubbed and cored
1 can (6½ ounces) water-packed tuna, drained (see note)
1 large egg, hard-cooked, peeled, and coarsely chopped
1 stalk celery, without leaves, scrubbed and finely chopped

1 large green onion, scrubbed, peeled, and finely chopped
¼ cup Delicious Homemade Mayonnaise (page 145)
Garlic powder to taste
Chopped fresh basil and dillweed to taste
2 tablespoons ground fresh almonds (optional)

Place lettuce leaves on 2 salad plates. Cut tomatoes into flowers by making 4–6 cuts from each center to bottom; pull "petals" away from center. Place tomato flowers on lettuce leaves. Mix tuna, egg, celery, green onion, mayonnaise, and seasonings in a small bowl. Spoon mixture equally into the center of each flower; press petals against filling. Top with almonds; chill before serving.

11 carbohydrates per serving

Note: Chicken may be used instead of tuna, if desired.

Guacamole Mold

SERVES 8 AS A SALAD, MORE AS AN APPETIZER

This is a unique and delicious salad mold or appetizer.

4 medium avocados, scrubbed, peeled, pitted, and quartered
1 medium yellow onion, scrubbed, peeled, and quartered
1 large tomato, scrubbed and quartered
¼ cup coarsely chopped fresh cilantro, rinsed and dried before chopping
2 teaspoons garlic powder
½ teaspoon sea salt (optional)
Cayenne pepper to taste
½ cup cold water (purified, preferably)
2 tablespoons Agar-Agar
¼ cup fresh lemon juice
1¾ cups boiling water (purified, preferably)

Blend avocados in food processor or with electric mixer until smooth. Transfer to a large bowl; cover. Place onion, tomato, and seasonings in processor; mix. Pour cold water into a small bowl. Add Agar-Agar; stir until dissolved. Add lemon juice; stir. Add boiling water to Agar; mix well. Add tomato mixture to avocado; mix. Add cooled Agar mixture. Place into a large, greased mold; chill until set. Serve with tortilla chips.

8 carbohydrates per salad serving

Marinated Buckwheat Salad

YIELDS 4 SERVINGS

Delicious buckwheat, vegetables, and fresh seasonings make a tasty salad. Caution: This is high in carbohydrates.

½ cup raw buckwheat
1 cup boiling water (purified, preferably)
¼ cup 100% pure, cold-pressed olive oil
¼ cup fresh lemon juice
2 large cloves garlic, scrubbed, peeled, and minced
3 small green onions, scrubbed, peeled, and chopped
1 large tomato, scrubbed and diced

1 medium lemon, scrubbed and chopped
2 tablespoons coarsely chopped fresh parsley
1 tablespoon coarsely chopped fresh mint
Sea salt to taste (optional)
4 large lettuce leaves, scrubbed and dried

Place buckwheat in a large mixing bowl; cover with boiling water. Let stand 1 hour; drain. Place buckwheat in a large bowl, adding all other ingredients, except lettuce leaves. Blend well. Cover and refrigerate 1–2 hours before serving, to allow flavors to blend. Spoon over lettuce leaves.

35 carbohydrates per serving

Savory Spanish Salad

YIELDS 4 SERVINGS

This delicious salad recipe, courtesy of Ida W. Klinger, Albuquerque, New Mexico will have your guests asking for the recipe!

1 medium cucumber, scrubbed, peeled, and diced
1 medium red bell pepper, scrubbed and diced
1 stalk celery, without leaves, scrubbed and chopped
3 small green onions, scrubbed, peeled, and chopped

2 tablespoons raw sunflower kernels (see note)
2 cups scrubbed, dried, and shredded romaine lettuce
4 ounces tortilla chips, crushed

Place all ingredients in a large salad bowl; toss with dressing (next page).

11 carbohydrates; 10 without sunflower kernels

Savory Spanish Dressing

YIELDS 4 SERVINGS

*1 medium avocado, scrubbed,
   peeled, pitted, and quartered*
*1 large fresh tomato, scrubbed
   and quartered*
*2 large green onions, scrubbed,
   peeled, and cut in half*

½ teaspoon garlic powder
2 tablespoons fresh lemon juice
Cayenne pepper to taste

Mix all ingredients in a food processor until creamy; pour over salad.

6 carbohydrates per serving

Note: If your digestive system is sensitive, omit the sunflower kernels.

Shrimp-Stuffed Avocado

YIELDS 2 SERVINGS

Your family or guests will relish this elegant salad.

*2 large lettuce leaves,
   scrubbed and dried*
*1 medium avocado, scrubbed,
   pitted, and halved*
*¼ pound cooked baby shrimp,
   rinsed (see note)*
*2 stalks celery, without leaves,
   scrubbed and finely chopped*
*2 small green onions, scrubbed,
   peeled, and finely chopped*

*¼ cup slivered or ground fresh
   almonds (see note)*
*2 tablespoons Delicious Home-
   made Mayonnaise (page 145)*
½ teaspoon chopped fresh basil
*1 medium fresh lemon,
   scrubbed and cut into wedges*

Place lettuce leaves on 2 salad plates. Top each leaf with an avocado half; cover with clear wrap. Mix the rest of the ingredients, minus the lemon, in a large bowl. Uncover avocado halves; fill with shrimp mixture; garnish with lemon wedges.

10 carbohydrates per serving

Note: Fresh crab may be used instead of shrimp if you wish. Substitute ground nuts for slivered if your digestive system is sensitive, or omit.

Spinach and Egg Salad

YIELDS 4 SERVINGS

You'll love to serve this colorful and tasty salad! Sweet Hot or Cold Tarragon Dressing (page 147) is a perfect accompaniment.

½ pound fresh spinach leaves, cleaned and dried

2 cups scrubbed and thinly sliced zucchini

1 medium yellow bell pepper, scrubbed and thinly sliced

1 medium red bell pepper, scrubbed and thinly sliced

8 cherry tomatoes, scrubbed and halved

1 can (2.2 ounces) sliced ripe olives, drained (optional)

2 large eggs, hard-cooked, peeled, and chopped

Tear spinach into bite-size pieces; place on 4 salad plates. Spread zucchini over spinach. Place yellow and red peppers at random. Sprinkle tomatoes and olives over tops. Cover with chopped eggs. Chill for 30 minutes to 1 hour before serving.

7 carbohydrates per serving

Sumi Oriental Salad

YIELDS 4 SERVINGS

This savory salad, courtesy of Raisa Sullivan, San Francisco, California.

1 green cabbage (approximately 3 pounds), scrubbed and shredded
½ package (2.5 ounces) bifun (Chinese noodles), cooked and drained

3 small green onions, scrubbed, peeled, and finely chopped
¼ cup slivered or ground fresh almonds (see note)
¼ cup sesame seeds, toasted

Mix all ingredients in a large bowl. Reserve for dressing below.

22 carbohydrates per serving

Sumi Dressing

½ cup cold-pressed sesame oil
¼ cup fresh lemon juice
2 tablespoons 100% Pure Vegetable Glycerine

½ tablespoon finely chopped scrubbed fresh gingerroot
½ teaspoon sea salt (optional)

Combine all ingredients in a small bowl, mix. Pour over salad; chill before serving.

4 carbohydrates per serving

Note: If your digestive system is sensitive, grind the nuts or omit.

Super Salmon Salad

YIELDS 2 SERVINGS

This is a good-tasting, easy salad for hot-weather meals.

1 can (7½ ounces) water-packed salmon, drained

2 stalks celery, without leaves, scrubbed and diced

2 small green onions, scrubbed, peeled, and coarsely chopped

½ cup frozen peas, cooked and cooled

1 large egg, hard-cooked, peeled, and chopped

1 can (2.2 ounces) sliced ripe olives, drained (optional)

2 tablespoons Delicious Home-made Mayonnaise (page 145)

1 tablespoon chopped fresh basil

2 large lettuce leaves, scrubbed and dried

Mix all ingredients, except lettuce leaves, in a large bowl. Place lettuce leaves on 2 salad plates. Spoon salad onto each leaf. Refrigerate at least 1 hour before serving.

20 carbohydrates per serving

Turkey and Quinoa Salad

YIELDS 4 SERVINGS

Quinoa makes a pleasing salad in combination with turkey or chicken.

½ cup raw quinoa
1 cup water (purified, preferably)
½ pound cooked natural turkey, cubed
3 small green onions, scrubbed, peeled, and coarsely chopped
⅓ cup 100% pure, cold-pressed olive oil

¼ cup fresh lemon juice
Curry powder to taste
Coarsely chopped fresh basil to taste
½ cup chopped or ground fresh pecans (see note)
4 large lettuce leaves, scrubbed and dried

Rinse quinoa well; drain. Place quinoa and water in a 2-quart saucepan; bring to a boil, then simmer, uncovered, for 10 minutes, or until all of the water is absorbed; cool. Place quinoa and all other ingredients, except lettuce leaves, in a large bowl; mix. Refrigerate 1–2 hours to allow flavors to blend. Spoon mixture onto lettuce leaves.

22 carbohydrates per serving

Note: If your digestive system is sensitive, try grinding the nuts or omit altogether.

Wild Rice Medley Salad

YIELDS 4 SERVINGS

Avocado and Lemon-Herb Dressing is used here to make a savory salad. Caution: This is somewhat high in carbohydrates.

1 cup cooked wild rice, cooled
2 cups scrubbed and shredded red cabbage
½ cup scrubbed and chopped fresh broccoli tops
½ medium red bell pepper, scrubbed and diced

½ cup chopped or ground fresh cashews (see note)
¼ cup raw sunflower kernels (see note)
Avocado and Lemon-Herb Dressing (page 143)

Blend all ingredients, except dressing, in a large bowl. Add enough dressing to coat ingredients well; toss. Refrigerate 1 hour before serving.

24 carbohydrates per serving; 22 without sunflower kernels

Note: If your digestive system is sensitive, you'll find that ground cashews are easier to digest than chopped. Also, omit sunflower kernels if you have digestive problems.

Avocado and Lemon-Herb Dressing

YIELDS APPROXIMATELY 3¾ CUPS

This outstanding salad dressing, courtesy of Nina Baker, Marin County, California, is a perfect accompaniment to spinach salad (see page 139) and all other green salads.

1 medium avocado, scrubbed, peeled, pitted, and quartered
2 cups pure, cold-pressed safflower oil
½ cup water (purified, preferably)
¼ cup fresh lemon juice
2 tablespoons each chopped fresh basil and parsley

1 tablespoon each chopped fresh oregano, thyme, tarragon, and savory
1 teaspoon each chopped fresh sage and rosemary
1 teaspoon sea salt (optional)

Place avocado in a blender or food processor; blend until creamy. Add rest of ingredients; blend until you have a liquid consistency. Pour dressing into a quart jar with a tight-fitting lid; refrigerate until ready to serve.

18 carbohydrates; 1 per tablespoon

Basil and Garlic Salad Oil

YIELDS APPROXIMATELY 1 CUP

This marvelously flavored salad oil enhances avocado, all green salads, and vegetables.

1 cup 100% pure, cold-pressed olive oil
6 stems fresh basil, with leaves

4 large cloves garlic, scrubbed, peeled, and coarsely chopped
¼ cup fresh lemon juice

Pour olive oil into a salad dressing cruet or 1-cup jar. Scrub basil; pull off leaves from stems and place in the oil. Add garlic. Cover with a tight-fitting lid; set on a sunny windowsill. Keep container there 2–7 days; for more flavor, leave longer. Shake container daily; taste for desired flavor. When ready, strain liquid carefully into a measuring cup; discard leaves and garlic. Pour liquid back into container; add lemon juice. Chill before serving.

9 carbohydrates; 1 per tablespoon

Creamy Herb Dressing

YIELDS APPROXIMATELY 1 CUP

This savory dressing is a delicious accompaniment to any salad.

½ cup pure, cold-pressed safflower oil
1 large tomato, scrubbed and quartered
¼ cup fresh lemon juice
2 large cloves garlic, peeled and crushed

½ teaspoon sea salt (optional)
1 tablespoon each chopped fresh thyme and tarragon
½ teaspoon ground paprika .
2 tablespoons 100% Pure Vegetable Glycerine
2 tablespoons sesame seeds

Place all ingredients in a blender, food processor, or wide-mouthed jar; mix well. Refrigerate before serving.

18 carbohydrates; 1 per tablespoon

Note: Refrigerate any leftover dressing in a jar with a tight-fitting lid.

Delicious Homemade Mayonnaise
YIELDS APPROXIMATELY 3 CUPS

This mayonnaise recipe will be your favorite!

6 large egg yolks
2 cups pure, cold-pressed
*   safflower oil*
1/4 cup fresh lemon juice

1/4 cup water (purified, preferably)
1 teaspoon sea salt (optional)
1 teaspoon dry mustard

Beat yolks for 2 minutes in a food processor or with an electric mixer. Pour 1 cup of the oil into a measuring cup. Very slowly drizzle a thin stream of oil from the cup into the yolks, while beating at high speed, until all has been used; mixture should become thick. Drizzle in remaining cup, still beating at high speed. Add lemon juice, water, salt, and mustard; mix. Mayonnaise is ready! Spoon mixture into a wide-mouthed quart jar with a tight-fitting lid. Refrigerate until ready to use.

1 carbohydrate per each 1/2 cup

Italian Dressing and Marinade

YIELDS APPROXIMATELY 1 CUP

This is a perfect recipe for marinating vegetables. Use it in Marinated Artichokes (page 122) as well as Baked Chicken Thighs with Artichokes and Almonds (page 83).

¼ cup fresh lemon juice
¼ cup water (purified,
  preferably)
⅓ cup 100% pure, cold-
  pressed olive oil
2 large cloves garlic,
  scrubbed, peeled, and
  minced

¼ teaspoon sea salt (optional)
1 tablespoon each coarsely
  chopped fresh oregano,
  basil, and sage

Place all ingredients in a pint jar with a tight-fitting lid; refrigerate at least 2–4 hours to allow flavors to blend. Shake well before serving.

7 carbohydrates; 0 per tablespoon

Poppy Seed French Dressing

YIELDS APPROXIMATELY 1 CUP

This lovely salad dressing combines glycerine, a permitted sweetener, with delicious herbs and poppy seeds.

½ cup pure, cold-pressed
  safflower oil
¼ cup fresh lemon juice
1 large clove garlic, scrubbed,
  peeled, and minced
½ teaspoon sea salt (optional)
½ teaspoon chopped fresh basil

1 teaspoon each chopped fresh
  thyme and tarragon
½ teaspoon ground paprika
2 tablespoons 100% Pure Vege-
  table Glycerine
¼ cup poppy seeds

Combine all ingredients in a blender or food processor; mix well. Refrigerate, covered, at least 1 hour before serving.

17 carbohydrates; 1 per tablespoon

Note: Refrigerate any leftover dressing in a jar with a tight-fitting lid.

Sweet Hot or Cold Tarragon Dressing
YIELDS APPROXIMATELY 2 CUPS

This unique and savory salad dressing is especially delicious when served hot over Spinach and Egg Salad (page 139). It is also tasty when chilled and served over any green salad.

2 tablespoons cold-pressed sesame oil
2 tablespoons scrubbed, peeled, and chopped white onion
½ can (8¾ ounces) Hain's unsweetened chicken broth
2 tablespoons 100% Pure Vegetable Glycerine

1 tablespoon fresh lemon juice
2 tablespoons chopped fresh tarragon
½ teaspoon dry mustard
1 tablespoon arrowroot powder
¼ cup water (purified, preferably)

Place sesame oil and onion in a large nonstick skillet; sauté until tender. Mix in broth, glycerine, lemon juice, tarragon, and mustard. Bring to a boil, then reduce heat to simmer. Mix arrowroot with water; pour into broth and mix until thick. Serve hot or cold.

14 carbohydrates; 1 per tablespoon

Note: Refrigerate any leftover dressing in a jar with a tight-fitting lid.

Thousand Island Dressing

YIELDS APPROXIMATELY ¾ CUP

This delicious salad dressing is a perfect accompaniment to seafood salads.

*½ cup Delicious Homemade
  Mayonnaise (page 00)*
1 tablespoon fresh lemon juice
*1 tablespoon unsweetened tomato
  sauce (without citric acid)*

*¼ medium red bell pepper,
  scrubbed and finely chopped*
*1 teaspoon scrubbed, peeled, and
  grated yellow onion*
1 tablespoon chopped fresh basil

Mix all ingredients in a small bowl. Chill 1 hour before serving to allow flavors to blend.

5 carbohydrates

Note: Refrigerate any leftover dressing in a jar with a tight-fitting lid.

Breads, Muffins, Rolls, Crepes, and Pancakes

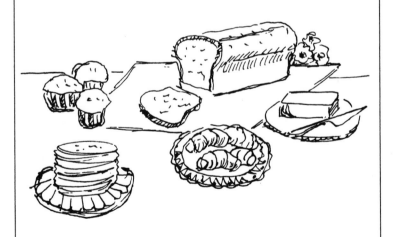

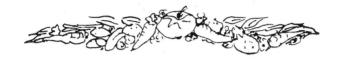

Mexicali Corn Bread

YIELDS NINE 2⅔-INCH PIECES

This marvelous corn bread can be served with any meal. Caution: It's high in carbohydrates.

1 cup cornmeal
½ cup each amaranth flour and millet flour
1 tablespoon baking powder
1 teaspoon sea salt (optional)
1 large egg
1 cup unsweetened soy milk (see note)
1 can (17 ounces) unsweetened corn, drained

¼ cup Easy Clarified Butter (page 37)
1 medium yellow onion, scrubbed, peeled, and chopped
1 small fresh green chili, scrubbed and chopped
1 medium red bell pepper, scrubbed and chopped
Cayenne pepper to taste

Preheat oven to 400°F. Place first 7 ingredients into a large bowl. Melt butter in a small skillet; add last 4 ingredients and cook until tender. Combine with bowl ingredients; mix. Pour into a greased 8-inch baking dish. Bake 35–40 minutes. Test for doneness with a toothpick.

37 carbohydrates each

Note: If you're sensitive to soy, try nut milk or egg whites instead (see "Dairy Substitutes").

Poppy Seed and Orange Loaf

YIELDS 12 SLICES

A delicious combination. Any leftovers can be easily frozen.

2 large eggs
1¹/2 cups brown rice flour
2¹/2 teaspoons baking powder
1 cup unsweetened soy milk (see note)
¹/4 cup Easy Clarified Butter melted (page 37)
2 teaspoons special orange flavoring (see page 210)

¹/4 cup 100% Pure Vegetable Glycerine
¹/2 teaspoon sea salt (optional)
1 teaspoon ground nutmeg
4 tablespoons poppy seeds
¹/2 cup chopped or ground fresh walnuts (see note)

Preheat oven to 350°F. Beat eggs in a large bowl until light. Add all other ingredients, except poppy seeds and nuts; beat until well blended. Fold in poppy seeds and nuts. Pour into a greased and lightly floured 5 × 9-inch loaf pan. Bake 40–50 minutes. Loaf is done when a toothpick comes out clean. Cool before slicing.

30 carbohydrates each

Note: If you're sensitive to soy, use nut milk or egg white instead (see "Dairy Substitutes"). And if your digestive system is sensitive, try ground rather than chopped nuts.

Pumpkin and Pecan Loaf

YIELDS 12 SLICES

The marvelous pumpkin aroma and flavor makes this a delicious treat for breakfasts, dinners, or snacks.

2 large eggs, beaten
⅓ cup Easy Clarified Butter (page 37)
¼ cup 100% Pure Vegetable Glycerine
2 cups canned unsweetened pumpkin
1¼ cups brown rice flour

½ teaspoon sea salt (optional)
2 teaspoons baking powder
¼ teaspoon ground cloves
½ teaspoon each ground cinnamon, ginger, and nutmeg
½ cup chopped or ground fresh pecans (see note)

Preheat oven to 350°F. Mix all ingredients except nuts in a large bowl until well blended. Mix in pecans. Pour batter into a well-greased and lightly floured, 5 × 9-inch loaf pan. Bake 50–60 minutes. Test for doneness with a toothpick. Cool before slicing.

23 carbohydrates each

Note: Remember, ground nuts are easier to digest than chopped.

Round Caraway Bread

YIELDS 16 SLICES

The combination of caraway and brown rice flour makes a delicious bread.

1½ cups brown rice flour
1½ teaspoons baking powder
½ teaspoon baking soda
½ teaspoon sea salt (optional)
1 tablespoon caraway seeds
¾ cup + 2 tablespoons unsweetened soy milk (see note)

2 large eggs, lightly beaten
2 tablespoons Easy Clarified Butter (page 37)
1 tablespoon 100% Pure Vegetable Glycerine

Preheat oven to 375°F. Mix all ingredients in a large bowl. Place dough in a greased round, 8-inch baking pan; pat dough down until it fills pan evenly. Bake 20–30 minutes, or until well browned.

20 carbohydrates each

Note: If you're sensitive to soy, try nut milk or egg whites instead (see ''Dairy Substitutes'').

Zucchini-Nut Bread

YIELDS 12 SLICES

This bread is delicious for any meal, dessert, or snack. Caution: It's high in carbohydrates.

1 1/2 cups + 2 tablespoons brown rice flour
1 teaspoon baking powder
1/2 teaspoon baking soda
1/2 teaspoon sea salt (optional)
2 large eggs, beaten
1/4 cup Easy Clarified Butter (page 37)
1 teaspoon special vanilla flavoring (see page 210)

1/4 cup 100% Pure Vegetable Glycerine
2 teaspoons ground cinnamon
1/2 teaspoon ground nutmeg
1 pound zucchini, scrubbed and shredded
1 cup chopped or ground fresh walnuts (see notes)

Preheat oven to 350°F. Mix all ingredients, except zucchini and nuts, in a large bowl. Fold in zucchini and nuts; spoon mixture into a greased and floured 5 × 9-inch loaf pan. Bake 45–50 minutes. Test for doneness with a toothpick. Cool before slicing.

26 carbohydrates each

Note: If digestive system is sensitive, try ground nuts instead. Do not store this bread; freeze any leftovers.

Festive Pumpkin and Nut Muffins

YIELDS 1 DOZEN MUFFINS

These delicious muffins are ideal snacks and as additions to meals.

1 ⅛ cups brown rice flour
2 teaspoons baking powder
½ cup unsweetened soy milk (see note)
¾ cup canned unsweetened pumpkin
¼ cup Easy Clarified Butter (page 37)
1 large egg

1 tablespoon 100% Pure Vegetable Glycerine
1 teaspoon special orange flavoring (see page 210)
½ teaspoon sea salt (optional)
½ teaspoon each ground cinnamon, nutmeg, and cloves
½ cup chopped fresh walnuts (see note)

Preheat oven to 400°F. Place all ingredients, except nuts, in a large bowl; mix until well moistened. Fold in nuts, batter will be lumpy. Fill greased muffin or paper baking cups. Bake 18–20 minutes, test for doneness with a toothpick.

21 carbohydrates each

Note: If you're sensitive to soy, use nut milk or egg white instead (see "Dairy Substitutes"). And if your digestive system is sensitive, try ground nuts instead of chopped.

Oat and Orange Muffins

YIELDS 1 DOZEN MUFFINS

Special orange flavoring is delightful when combined with oat bran.

2 cups oat bran cereal
2 teaspoons baking powder
1/2 teaspoon sea salt (optional)
1 cup unsweetened soy milk (see note)
2 large eggs, beaten
2 tablespoons Easy Clarified Butter (page 37)

1/4 cup 100% Pure Vegetable Glycerine
2 teaspoons special orange flavoring (see page 210)
1/4 cup chopped or ground fresh walnuts (see note)

Preheat oven to 400°F. Place all ingredients in a large bowl; mix until well blended. Batter will be lumpy. Spoon batter into greased muffin or paper baking cups, filling ⅔ full. Bake 15–18 minutes. Test for doneness with a toothpick.

15 carbohydrates each

Note: If you're sensitive to soy, nut milk or egg whites may be used instead (see "Dairy Substitutes"). If your digestive system is sensitive, ground nuts are easier to digest than chopped.

Sunny Corn Muffins

YIELDS 1 DOZEN MUFFINS

How wonderful to wake up to these delightful muffins! They are also a great treat for other meals or snacks.

1 cup yellow cornmeal
1/2 cup each amaranth flour and millet flour
1 tablespoon baking powder
1 teaspoon sea salt (optional)
1 tablespoon 100% Pure Vegetable Glycerine

1 cup unsweetened soy milk (see note)
1/3 cup Easy Clarified Butter (page 37)
1 large egg, beaten

Preheat oven to 400°F. Place all ingredients in a large bowl; mix. Pour batter into greased muffin or paper baking cups, filling them ⅔ full. Bake 15–20 minutes. Use the toothpick test to determine doneness. Serve warm with Easy Clarified Butter if you like.

23 carbohydrates each

Note: If you're sensitive to soy, try nut milk or egg whites instead (see "Dairy Substitutes"). This recipe also makes delicious corn bread. Prepare in the same manner and bake in a greased 8-inch baking dish.

Caraway Rolls

YIELDS 2 DOZEN ROLLS

Caraway, brown rice flour, dairy substitutes, and glycerine sweetener make delicious rolls.

2½ cups sifted brown rice flour
2 teaspoons baking powder
½ teaspoon baking soda
½ teaspoon sea salt (optional)
¾ cup + 2 tablespoons unsweetened soy milk (see note)

1 large egg, lightly beaten
2 tablespoons Easy Clarified Butter (page 37), melted
1 tablespoon 100% Pure Vegetable Glycerine
2 tablespoons caraway seeds

Preheat oven to 375°F. Mix all ingredients, except caraway seeds, in a large bowl; until well blended. For narrow, oblong rolls, roll small pieces of dough into capsule shapes; roll in caraway seeds. For Parker House roll shape, pat dough (on a floured board) into an oval shape, measuring approximately 2½ × 1½ inches. Fold one side over to other side. Roll in caraway seeds. Place on a nonstick baking sheet; bake 15 minutes.

21 carbohydrates each

Note: If you're sensitive to soy, nut milk or egg whites may be used instead (see "Dairy Substitutes").

Cinnamon and Nut Rolls

YIELDS 1 DOZEN ROLLS

Delicious sweet rolls made with 100% Pure Vegetable Glycerine. Caution: These are high in carbohydrates.

1¾ cups brown rice flour
1 tablespoon baking powder
½ teaspoon sea salt (optional)
2 tablespoons Easy Clarified Butter (page 37)
⅔ cup unsweetened soy milk (see note)
1 tablespoon 100% Pure Vegetable Glycerine

1 teaspoon ground cinnamon
Cinnamon-Nut Topping (page 196)
1 tablespoon 100% Pure Vegetable Glycerine
1 teaspoon ground cinnamon

Preheat oven to 400°F. Place first 7 ingredients into a large bowl; mix with pastry blender, fork, or 2 knives. Form dough into a ball. Place dough on a floured board. Roll, with a floured rolling pin, into a ¼-inch thick rectangle. Spread topping over dough. Roll up lengthwise; cut into ¾-inch slices. Butter an 8-inch round cake pan; sprinkle remaining glycerine and cinnamon on bottom of pan. Place rolls on top. Bake 10–15 minutes. ⸴

30 carbohydrates each

Note: If you're sensitive to soy, nut milk or egg white may be used instead (see "Dairy Substitutes").

Popovers

YIELDS 1 DOZEN POPOVERS

These delicious popovers, with their marvelous texture, are especially enjoyable when served hot, with dabs of melted clarified butter.

4 large eggs
¾ cup brown rice flour
1 cup unsweetened soy milk (see note)

½ teaspoon sea salt (optional)
1 tablespoon Easy Clarified Butter (page 37), melted

Preheat oven to 400°F. Place all ingredients in a large bowl; beat until well blended. Generously grease muffin or paper baking cups. Spoon batter evenly into cups. Bake 30 minutes, or until puffed and browned. Serve immediately.

17 carbohydrates each

Note: If you're sensitive to soy, nut milk or egg whites may be used instead (see "Dairy Substitutes").

Poppy Seed and Herb Biscuits
YIELDS 1 DOZEN BISCUITS

The combination of poppy seeds and thyme makes these biscuits delightful, especially when served warm.

1¼ cups brown rice flour, unsifted
1 tablespoon baking powder
1 tablespoon poppy seeds
½ teaspoon sea salt (optional)
⅓ cup Easy Clarified Butter (page 37), melted

¾ cup unsweetened soy milk (see note)
1 large egg, beaten
1 teaspoon chopped fresh thyme

Preheat oven to 375°F. Place all ingredients in a large bowl; mix until smooth. Place dough by the tablespoonful on a nonstick baking sheet, either 1-inch apart (for crisp ends) or touching (for soft ends). Bake 15–18 minutes, testing for doneness with a toothpick. Serve warm with Easy Clarified Butter.

23 carbohydrates each

Note: If you're sensitive to soy, try nut milk or egg whites instead (see "Dairy Substitutes").

Sesame Rolls Royale

YIELDS 1 DOZEN ROLLS

These rolls are a delicious treat for guests; freeze them and use as needed. Caution: they're high in carbohydrates.

*2 tablespoons Easy Clarified
  Butter (page 37)*
¼ cup sesame seeds
1¾ cups brown rice flour
1 tablespoon baking powder

½ teaspoon sea salt (optional)
*⅔ cup unsweetened soy milk (see
  note)*
2 large eggs

Preheat oven to 400°F. Melt butter in a small skillet. Add sesame seeds; sauté until lightly browned; cool and reserve. Meanwhile, mix flour, baking powder, and salt in a large bowl. Add milk. Separate eggs; beat egg whites until thick and fold into flour mixture. Roll dough into 2-inch balls; flatten. Stir yolks; dip rolls into yolks; then into sesame seeds. Place on a nonstick baking sheet. Bake 15–17 minutes, testing for doneness with a toothpick.

31 carbohydrates each

Note: Try nut milk or egg whites if you're sensitive to soy (see "Dairy Substitutes").

Sweet Orange Rolls

YIELDS 1 DOZEN ROLLS

Orange flavoring and other fine substitutes show off! Caution: This is high in carbohydrates.

1¾ cups brown rice flour
1 tablespoon baking powder
½ teaspoon sea salt
*2 tablespoons Easy Clarified Butter
  (page 37)*
*⅔ cup unsweetened soy milk (see
  note)*
*2 tablespoons 100% Pure
  Vegetable Glycerine*

*2 teaspoons special orange
  flavoring (see page 210)*
*2 tablespoons Easy Clarified
  Butter*
1 tablespoon Vegetable Glyercine
*1 teaspoon special orange
  flavoring*
½ cup ground fresh pecans

Preheat oven to 400°F. Mix first 7 ingredients in a large bowl until well blended. Form dough into a ball; roll out to a rectangle 1/8-inch thick. Mix 2 more tablespoons melted butter, glycerine, flavoring and nuts. Spread over dough; roll up and cut into 3/4-inch pieces. Place on a nonstick baking sheet. Bake 10-15 minutes.

30 carbohydrates each

Note: If sensitive to soy, nut milk or egg whites may be used instead (see "Dairy Substitutes").

Tasty Crepes

YIELDS APPROXIMATELY 10 CREPES

These crepes are used for Cheese Blintzes (page 164), Chicken and Broccoli Crepes (page 162), and Spinach Crepes (page 162). Caution: They're high in carbohydrates.

3 large eggs
1 cup brown rice flour
1 1/2 cups unsweetened soy milk (see note)
1/2 teaspoon sea salt (optional)
1/2 tablespoon special vanilla flavoring (see page 210)

1 tablespoon 100% Pure Vegetable Glycerine
Easy Clarified Butter (page 37)

Lemon-Butter Sauce (page 178) (optional)

Using an electric mixer, beat eggs until light. Add flour, soy milk, salt, vanilla, and glycerine; beat 2 minutes at high speed. In a small nonstick skillet, melt enough butter to cover bottom of pan; heat to medium-high. When butter is hot, drop in a large spoonful of batter. Tilt pan back and forth to spread batter evenly. Turn crepe when lightly browned, then brown other side lightly. Place crepe on a serving plate. Repeat process; keep crepes warm in oven until serving. Serve with Lemon-Butter Sauce.

28 carbohydrates each

Note: If you're sensitive to soy, try nut milk or egg whites instead (see "Dairy Substitutes").

Chicken and Broccoli Crepes

YIELDS APPROXIMATELY 10 CREPES

This is a delicious entrée for meals or parties. Caution: It's high in carbohydrates.

4 chicken breast halves
water (purified preferably)
1 package (10 ounces) frozen
   broccoli, thawed and cooked

1 tablespoon yellow onion,
   scrubbed, peeled, and grated
1 teaspoon garlic powder
Tasty Crepes (page 161)

Preheat oven to 400°F. Place chicken breasts in a large skillet; add enough water to cover. Bring to a boil; simmer 15–20 minutes, or until tender. Drain broccoli; coarsely chop and place in a large bowl. Cool chicken; remove skin and bones. Coarsely chop chicken and add to broccoli. Add onion and garlic powder; mix. Spoon mixture over crepes; roll. Place crepes in a greased 8-inch baking dish. Bake covered 15–20 minutes.

29 carbohydrates each

Spinach Crepes

YIELDS 10 CREPES

These delicious crepes are elegant for entertaining. Caution: They're high in carbohydrates.

1 package (10 ounces) frozen
   chopped spinach, thawed
2 tablespoons 100% pure, cold-
   pressed olive oil
2 large cloves garlic, scrubbed,
   peeled, and minced

1 medium white onion,
   scrubbed, peeled, and chopped
Ground nutmeg to taste
Tasty Crepes (page 161)

Mock Sour Cream (page 197)

Preheat oven to 350°F. Squeeze out all liquid from spinach. Heat oil in a large skillet. Sauté garlic and onion until tender.

Add spinach and nutmeg to skillet mixture; turn and mix until spinach is well coated, and remove from heat. Place spinach mixture on the center of each crepe. Roll and place crepes into a large, greased casserole. Bake, covered, 20–30 minutes. Serve with Mock Sour Cream.

31 carbohydrates per serving

Baked German Pancake

YIELDS 4 SERVINGS

This delicious, huge pancake is a real treat for Sunday brunch. Lemon-Butter Sauce is a perfect accompaniment. Caution: It's high in carbohydrates.

1/4 cup Easy Clarified Butter (page 37)
4 large eggs
1/2 cup brown rice flour
1/2 teaspoon sea salt (optional)
1/2 cup unsweetened soy milk (see note)

1 teaspoon special vanilla flavoring (see page 210)
1 medium lemon, scrubbed and cut into wedges (optional)
Lemon-Butter Sauce (page 178) (optional)

Preheat oven to 450°F. Use butter to grease bottom and sides of an 8-inch iron skillet from which handle has been removed or an 8-inch round nonstick baking pan. Beat eggs until light in a large bowl, then add flour, salt, milk, and vanilla. Beat at high speed 2 minutes. Pour batter into skillet. Bake 18– 20 minutes, or until golden brown. Serve immediately with pats of butter and wedges of lemon or Lemon-Butter Sauce.

31 carbohydrates per serving

Note: If you're sensitive to soy, use nut milk or egg whites instead (see "Dairy Substitutes").

Cheese Blintzes (Filled Pancakes)

YIELDS APPROXIMATELY 10 BLINTZES

These delicious, cheese-filled pancakes are of Eastern European origin. Caution: They're high in carbohydrates.

1 large egg, beaten
1 cup raw cottage cheese (see note)
1 tablespoon 100% Pure Vegetable Glycerine

1 teaspoon ground cinnamon
Easy Clarified Butter (page 37)
Tasty Crepes (page 161)
Mock Sour Cream (page 40)

Mix all ingredients except butter, crepes, and sour cream in a small bowl. Spoon mixture evenly on the center of each pancake. Fold each side over and into an envelope shape. Melt enough butter to cover bottom of a large skillet. Fry each side of crepe 5 minutes over medium-high heat until golden brown. Serve with Mock Sour Cream.

30 carbohydrates each

Note: If your digestive system is sensitive, do not use raw cottage cheese; try fresh tofu or fill the crepes with spinach or chicken and broccoli (see page 162).

Potato Latkes (Pancakes)

YIELDS APPROXIMATELY 10 PANCAKES

These scrumptious pancakes use potato flour instead of wheat flour.

4 medium new potatoes
water (purified, preferably)
2 large eggs
1/2 teaspoon sea salt (optional)
1 tablespoon potato flour

1/8 teaspoon baking powder
1 medium yellow onion,
*   scrubbed, peeled, and grated*
Easy Clarified Butter (page 37)
Mock Sour Cream (page 40)

Scrub, peel, and immediately soak potatoes in a bowl of cold water. Beat eggs in another bowl. Add salt, flour, baking powder, and onion to eggs; mix. Drain potatoes; grate and add to eggs. Heat enough butter to cover bottom of a large nonstick skillet; drop in spoonfuls of batter. Brown on both sides. Serve with Mock Sour Cream.

10 carbohydrates each

Potato Kugel (pudding)

Instead of browning in a skillet, place the ingredients for latkes—except the butter—in a greased 8-inch baking dish. Melt enough butter and drizzle it over the top. Bake in a preheated 350°F oven for thirty minutes, or until brown. Serve with Mock Sour Cream (p. 197).

17 carbohydrates per 9-inch square piece

Wild Rice Pancakes

YIELDS 12 PANCAKES

These flavorful pancakes are a delicious change from the ordinary. Pancake Syrup Surprise is a perfect accompaniment. Caution: These are high in carbohydrates.

1 cup brown rice flour
1 tablespoon baking powder
1/4 teaspoon sea salt (optional)
1 large egg
1 cup unsweetened soy milk (see note)
2 tablespoons Easy Clarified Butter (page 37), melted

1 teaspoon 100% Pure Vegetable Glycerine
1/4 cup raw wild rice, cooked
Pancake Syrup Surprise (page 197)

Place flour, baking powder, and salt in a large bowl; blend. Beat egg and milk in another bowl until well blended. Add butter to egg mixture; mix and pour into flour mixture. Add glycerine and rice; mix well. Drop in spoonfuls onto a preheated, greased griddle or skillet; turn when brown. Brown other side; serve with Pancake Syrup Surprise.

23 carbohydrates each

Note: If you're sensitive to soy, try nut milk or egg whites instead (see ''Dairy Substitutes'').

Beverages

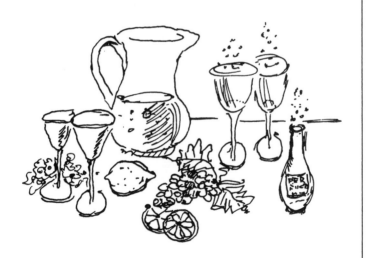

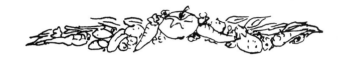

Perrier Cocktail

To feel really elegant, get out your best cocktail glasses and enjoy!

Chilled Perrier water
Lime or lemon, scrubbed and cut
* into wedges*

Pour Perrier into glass or glasses; garnish with lime or lemon.

0 carbohydrates

Note: You may ask for a Perrier Cocktail when dining out. Most waiters or hosts will be happy to oblige when you tell them how to do it.

Lemon Cooler

YIELDS 6 SERVINGS

This is a refreshing, delightful-tasting drink, using 100% Pure Vegetable Glycerine.

½ cup fresh lemon juice
1 quart water (purified, preferably)
¼ cup 100% Pure Vegetable Glycerine

3 cups ice cubes (purified water, preferably)
6 fresh mint leaves

Combine all ingredients in a large pitcher. Enjoy!

2 carbohydrates per serving

Mock Margaritas

YIELDS 2 SERVINGS

You can really celebrate with this delicious copy of the real thing.

5 fresh limes, scrubbed and cut in halves
Sea salt (optional)
1½ cups crushed ice (purified water, preferably)

2 tablespoons 100% Pure Vegetable Glycerine

Using 2 large Margarita or wine glasses, rub ½ lime around rims. Pour salt on a small, flat plate. Roll rims of glasses in salt. Squeeze juice of rest of limes into a blender, reserving ½ lime for garnish. Add ice and glycerine. Mix until foamy. Pour beverage into glasses. Cut reserved lime half into 2 wedges; garnish.

13 carbohydrates per serving

Carrot Delight

YIELDS 2 SERVINGS

This is not only a tasty drink, but healthful as well due to beta carotene, which is beneficial for *Candida*. A note of caution: This is high in carbohydrates.

6 carrots, scrubbed, peeled,
  and chopped into 2" pieces
1½ cups mineral water
1 tablespoon grated fresh
  gingerroot, or more, to taste

Ice cubes (made from purified
  water, preferably)

Place carrots in a blender or juicer. Add mineral water and ginger. Blend until liquid consistency. Add ice cubes; mix until crushed. (Beverage may be thick.) Pour mixture into two 8-ounce glasses and serve.

21 carbohydrates per serving

Cranberry Zinger

YIELDS 2 SERVINGS

Unsweetened cranberry concentrate makes an easy-to-prepare and refreshing thirst quencher.

2 cups mineral water
2 tablespoons unsweetened
  cranberry concentrate

Ice cubes (made from purified
  water, preferably)

Combine mineral water and cranberry concentrate in a blender. Add 6–8 ice cubes. Blend until mixture is foamy. Place 3–4 ice cubes in two 8-ounce glasses. Pour cranberry mixture into glasses and serve.

9 carbohydrates per serving

Note: There is no need to strain this drink.

Healthy Mary

YIELDS 2 SERVINGS

This non-alcoholic drink is delicious as well as nourishing. Enjoy!

2 large fresh tomatoes, scrubbed, peeled, and cored
Juice from 1 medium lemon, scrubbed before cutting
½ teaspoon celery seed, more or less, to taste
1 teaspoon sea salt (optional)

Dash cayenne pepper, or more, to taste
Ice cubes (made from purified water, preferably)
2 fresh lime wedges, scrubbed before cutting

Blend tomatoes in a food processor or blender until liquid consistency; strain and remove seeds. Add rest of ingredients, except lime; mix. Place ice cubes in two 8-ounce glasses, filling them ½ full. Pour tomato mixture over cubes. Squeeze a lime wedge into each glass; mix.

9 carbohydrates per serving

Iced Chamomile

YIELDS 2 SERVINGS

This delightful plan-ahead drink is perfect for lunch, dinner, or afternoon treat.

1½ cups water (purified, preferably), boiled
3 Chamomile tea bags
8–10 ice cubes (purified, preferably)

2 stems and leaves fresh mint, rinsed

Pour boiled water over tea bags. Let steep for 3 minutes; cool. Remove tea bags and place mixture into a blender. Add ice cubes. Blend just until foamy. Pour into two 8-ounce glasses. Garnish with mint.

0 carbohydrates per serving

Vegetable Spritzer

YIELDS 2–4 SERVINGS

This colorful and delicious drink will be a special treat for you. It may be served either chilled or heated. A note of caution: This is high in carbohydrates.

1 medium cucumber, scrubbed and peeled	*2 medium raw beets, without tops, scrubbed and peeled*
2 stalks celery, without leaves, scrubbed	*Juice from 2 medium lemons, scrubbed before cutting*
½ cup chopped parsley tops, rinsed before cutting	*½ teaspoon garlic powder*
½ green pepper, scrubbed before cutting, and seeded	*½ teaspoon sea salt*
½ medium onion, scrubbed before cutting, and peeled	*Ice cubes (made from purified water, preferably)*

Blend all ingredients except ice cubes in a blender or juicer until liquid consistency. Strain, if necessary. Pour into glasses, filled ½ full with ice cubes, and serve.

21 carbohydrates per serving for 2; 14 carbohydrates per serving for 3

Note: Instead of serving drink chilled, heat in a 2-quart saucepan over medium-high heat, until hot, and serve in cups.

Sauces

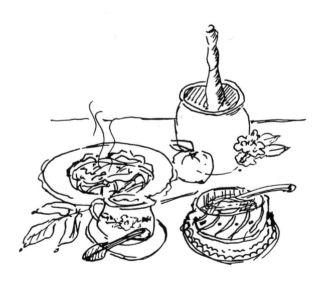

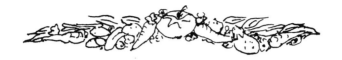

Easy Hollandaise Sauce

YIELDS APPROXIMATELY ½ CUP

This savory sauce gives ideal flavor to vegetables such as asparagus and broccoli.

½ cup Delicious Homemade   *1 large egg yolk*
  Mayonnaise (page 145)   *¼ teaspoon sea salt (optional)*
1 tablespoon fresh lemon juice   *Ground nutmeg to taste*

Place mayonnaise and lemon juice in a small nonstick saucepan. Add egg yolk and salt and continually stir with a whisk over medium-high heat. When hot, but not boiling, add nutmeg; stir. Remove from heat immediately; serve with or over vegetables.

2 carbohydrates

Lemon-Butter Sauce

YIELDS APPROXIMATELY ¾ CUP

This delicious sauce enhances brown rice, vegetables, fish, or chicken and is a delicious accompaniment to Tasty Crepes (page 161).

½ cup Easy Clarified Butter   *¼ cup fresh lemon juice*
(page 37)   *Sea salt to taste (optional)*

Melt butter in a small skillet. Add lemon juice and salt; mix. Remove from heat immediately. Serve sauce over crepes and other entrées or separately in a bowl to accompany them.

4 carbohydrates

Note: This sauce may also be used with sautéed chicken breasts; try adding fresh tarragon and garlic for delightful flavor.

Napoletana Sauce

YIELDS APPROXIMATELY 2¾ CUPS

This savory sauce may be served over cooked soba (pure buckwheat spaghetti) or corn noodles.

1 can (15 ounces) unsweetened tomato sauce (without citric acid)
1 can (6 ounces) tomato paste (without citric acid)
2 tablespoons 100% pure, cold-pressed olive oil

1 tablespoon each chopped fresh basil, oregano, and sage
1 teaspoon each garlic powder and onion powder

Place all ingredients in a 2-quart saucepan; bring to a boil. Reduce heat; simmer, uncovered, 20 minutes. Serve hot over pasta.

12 carbohydrates per ½ cup

Note: Refrigerate any leftover sauce in a jar with a tight-fitting lid.

Saucy Salsa

YIELDS APPROXIMATELY 2½ CUPS

This zesty sauce may be served with any Mexican dish or with tortilla chips.

2 large fresh tomatoes, scrubbed, peeled, cored, puréed, and strained
1 large clove garlic, scrubbed, peeled, and minced
2 tablespoons fresh lemon juice
2 tablespoons yellow onion, scrubbed, peeled, and coarsely chopped

1 scrubbed and coarsely chopped fresh chili pepper to taste
¼ cup chopped fresh cilantro, rinsed before cutting

Place tomatoes and garlic in a 2-quart saucepan; boil until tender. Remove from heat; cool. Beat in food processor or with electric mixer until sauce consistency. Add other ingredients; mix. Spoon sauce into a bowl and serve.

5 carbohydrates per ½ cup

Note: Refrigerate any leftover sauce in a jar with a tight-fitting lid.

Special Spaghetti Sauce

YIELDS APPROXIMATELY 4¼ CUPS

This flavorful sauce may be served with soba (pure buckwheat spaghetti) or corn noodles.

4 large fresh tomatoes, scrubbed,
peeled, cored, puréed, and
strained
1 tablespoon coarsely chopped
fresh basil
1 tablespoon each coarsely
chopped fresh oregano and sage

½ teaspoon celery salt
¼ cup 100% pure, cold-pressed
olive oil
2 large cloves garlic, scrubbed,
peeled, and minced

Place tomato purée in a 2-quart saucepan; bring to a boil and reduce heat; add seasonings. Heat oil in a small skillet. Add garlic, and stir, sautéeing until tender; add to tomatoes. Simmer, uncovered, 30 minutes. Cover; simmer for 30 minutes longer. Serve over or with soba.

3 carbohydrates per ½ cup

Tasty Tartar Sauce

YIELDS APPROXIMATELY ¾ CUP

This sauce is a perfect accompaniment to any fish or shellfish entrée.

½ cup Delicious Homemade
Mayonnaise (page 145)
½ medium cucumber, scrubbed,
peeled, and finely chopped
¼ medium yellow onion, scrubbed,
peeled, and finely chopped

¼ medium lemon, unpeeled,
scrubbed, and finely chopped
1 tablespoon chopped fresh
dillweed

Place all ingredients in a small bowl; mix well. Chill 1 hour before serving to allow flavors to blend.

9 carbohydrates

Desserts

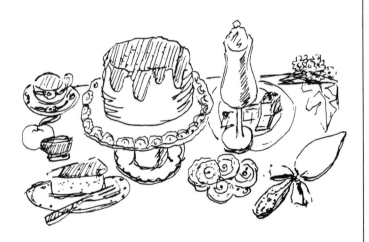

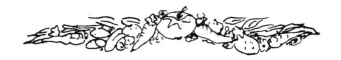

Best Poppy Seed Cake

YIELDS 10 SERVINGS

Clever substitutions make our family's favorite cake a delicious success! Caution: This plan-ahead recipe is high in carbohydrates.

1/4 cup + 2 tablespoons poppy seeds
1/4 cup + 2 tablespoons unsweetened soy milk (see note)
3/4 cup brown rice flour
1/2 cup arrowroot powder
1 teaspoon baking powder
1/4 cup Easy Clarified Butter (page 37)

3 tablespoons 100% Pure Vegetable Glycerine
1 teaspoon special vanilla flavoring (see page 210)
2 large eggs
Pecan Custard Topping (page 198)

Mix poppy seeds with milk in a small bowl; cover and soak 4–6 hours. Preheat oven to 375°F. Mix arrowroot powder, baking powder, butter, glycerine, flour, and vanilla flavoring in a large bowl. Separate eggs. Beat yolks; add to mixture. Beat whites until they form stiff peaks. Fold whites and poppy seed mixture into flour mixture. Pour batter into a well-greased, 8-inch square or round cake pan. Bake 20 minutes. Test for doneness with a toothpick; cool. Spread with topping.

28 carbohydrates per serving

Note: If you're sensitive to soy, nut milk or egg whites may be used instead (see "Dairy Substitutes").

Lemon Cake Supreme

YIELDS 10 SERVINGS

This egg-rich cake is elegant, and Almond and Butter Cream Icing is the perfect topping. Caution: It's high in carbohydrates.

1¹/2 cups brown rice flour
2 tablespoons arrowroot powder
1 tablespoon baking powder
6 large eggs
¹/2 cup Easy Clarified Butter (page 37), melted
¹/3 cup fresh lemon juice

1 tablespoon special lemon flavoring (see page 210)
5 tablespoons 100% Pure Vegetable Glycerine
Almond and Butter Cream Icing (page 196)

Preheat oven to 350°F. Mix flour, arrowroot powder, and baking powder in a large bowl. Separate eggs; beat yolks in another bowl with electric mixer until light. Add butter, lemon juice, flavoring, and glycerine to yolks, mix well and add to flour mixture. Beat until smooth. Beat egg whites until stiff; fold into flour mixture. Pour batter into a greased and lightly floured bundt or angel food cake pan. Bake 35–40 minutes. Test for doneness with a toothpick. When cool, may spread with icing, or cake is delicious plain.

30 carbohydrates per serving with icing; 29 carbohydrates without

Delightful Cheesecake

YIELDS 6 SERVINGS

Yes, it is even possible to have cheesecake on the diet!

1¹/2 cups raw cottage cheese (see note)
1 cup plain low-fat yogurt
3 large eggs
¹/4 cup 100% Pure Vegetable Glycerine

1 tablespoon arrowroot powder
1 teaspoon special vanilla flavoring (see page 210)
2 tablespoons fresh lemon juice
Perfect Pecan Crust (page 193)

Preheat oven to 350°F. Blend cottage cheese and yogurt in a food processor or electric mixer until smooth. Beat in eggs, one at a time. Add glycerine, arrowroot, vanilla, and lemon juice; mix well. Pour into Perfect Pecan Crust; bake 25 minutes. Turn oven off and open door, leaving cheesecake inside for 1 hour. Cool; refrigerate 2–3 hours before serving.

9 carbohydrates per serving

Note: If you have digestive problems, do not use raw cottage cheese; try fresh tofu, if you know you tolerate it.

Nutty Tofu Cheesecake

YIELDS 6 SERVINGS

The pleasant, nutty flavor makes a delightful cheesecake.

1¹/2 pounds fresh tofu
1/4 cup Easy Clarified Butter
(page 37), melted
2 tablespoons 100% Pure
Vegetable Glycerine
2 tablespoons fresh lemon juice
1/4 cup unsweetened soy milk (see note)

1/2 tablespoon special vanilla flavoring (see page 210)
1/4 teaspoon sea salt (optional)
Perfect Pecan Crust (page 193)
1/2 cup chopped or ground fresh pecans (see note)

Preheat oven to 325°F. Placed tofu in a colander, pressing with a fork to drain completely. Mix tofu and other ingredients (except crust and nuts), using a food processor or electric mixer, until smooth. Spoon mixture into Perfect Pecan Crust; top with nuts. Bake 1 hour; remove from oven. Let stand 30 minutes. Cover; refrigerate 2 hours before serving.

10 carbohydrates per serving

Note: If you're sensitive to soy, nut milk or egg whites may be used instead (see "Dairy Substitutes"). If your digestive system is sensitive, try using ground nuts instead of chopped, or omit altogether.

Festive Carrot Cookies

YIELDS 2 DOZEN COOKIES

Delicious cookies for special occasions or an anytime treat.

1/2 cup raw oat bran
1/2 cup brown rice flour
2 carrots, scrubbed, peeled, and
   finely chopped
1/4 cup Easy Clarified Butter
   (page 37), melted
2 tablespoons 100% Pure Vege-
   table Glycerine

1 large egg
1/2 cup chopped or ground
   fresh pecans (see note)
1 teaspoon special vanilla
   flavoring (see page 210)
1/4 teaspoon sea salt (optional)
2 teaspoons ground cinnamon

Preheat oven to 350°F. Place all ingredients in a large bowl; mix well. Place spoonfuls on a non-stick cookie sheet. Flatten with back of spoon. Bake 10–12 minutes.

6 carbohydrates each

Note: If your digestive system is sensitive, try ground nuts rather than chopped, or omit altogether.

Lemon and Pecan Cookies

YIELDS 2 DOZEN COOKIES

Lemon flavoring and pecans are a delicious combination in these delightful cookies.

1/2 cup Easy Clarified Butter
   (page 37), melted
3 tablespoons 100% Pure Vege-
   table Glycerine
1 large egg
1 1/2 cups + 4 1/2 teaspoons brown
   rice flour

1/2 teaspoon baking soda
1/4 cup fresh lemon juice
2 tablespoons special lemon
   flavoring (see page 210)
1/2 cup chopped or ground
   pecans (see note)

Preheat oven to 375°F. Mix butter and glycerine in a large bowl. Add egg, flour, and baking soda; mix well. Fold in lemon juice, flavoring, and pecans. Drop rounded teaspoonfuls of dough onto a nonstick cookie sheet. Bake 8–10 minutes. Cool 5 minutes before removing from cookie sheet.

12 carbohydrates each

Note: Try ground nuts rather than chopped if your digestive system is sensitive, or omit altogether.

Nut Butter Cookies

YIELDS 4 DOZEN COOKIES

These cookies are delicious and can be easily frozen.

1/4 cup Easy Clarified Butter (page 37), melted
1/2 cup Delicious and Easy Nut Butter (page 37)
2 tablespoons 100% Pure Vegetable Glycerine
1/3 cup unsweetened soy milk (see note)
1 large egg

1 teaspoon special vanilla flavoring (see page 210)
1 1/4 cups sifted brown rice flour
1 teaspoon baking powder
1/4 teaspoon sea salt (optional)
2 dozen fresh pecans or walnuts (see note), cut into halves or ground

Preheat oven to 350°F. Combine butters, glycerine, milk, egg, and flavoring in a large bowl. Place dry ingredients in another large bowl; mix together. Add dry mixture to milk mixture; blend well. Place teaspoonfuls of dough on a nonstick cookie sheet; flatten cookies with back of spoon; press nut halves into tops. Bake 8–10 minutes. Let cookies cool for 5 minutes before removing them from cookie sheet. Cookies will harden as they cool.

5 carbohydrates each

Note: Try nut milk or egg whites if you're sensitive to soy (see "Dairy Substitutes"). If your digestive system is sensitive, use ground nuts, or omit altogether.

Oat and Nut Cookies

YIELDS 2 DOZEN COOKIES

These cookies are a delicious treat and can be made ahead of time and frozen for unexpected guests or as snacks.

1 cup + 2 tablespoons raw oat bran
1/2 cup brown rice flour
3/8 cup Easy Clarified Butter (page 37), melted
2 tablespoons 100% Pure Vegetable Glycerine
1 large egg

1/2 teaspoon special vanilla flavoring (see page 210)
1/2 teaspoon sea salt (optional)
1/4 teaspoon baking soda
1/2 teaspoon ground cinnamon
1/2 cup chopped or ground fresh walnuts (see note)

Preheat oven to 350°F. Place all ingredients in a large bowl; mix well. Form 1-inch balls; place on a nonstick cookie sheet. Flatten with back of spoon. Bake 8–10 minutes or until golden brown. Let cookies cool on cookie sheet for 5 minutes; cookies will harden as they cool.

7 carbohydrates each

Note: Try ground nuts rather than chopped if your digestive system is sensitive, or omit altogether.

Pumpkin Cookies

YIELDS 3 DOZEN COOKIES

The delightful flavor combination of pumpkin and orange makes these cookies a welcome treat.

*1 cup canned unsweetened
   pumpkin*
*1/2 cup Easy Clarified Butter
   (page 37), melted*
*1/4 cup 100% Pure Vegetable
   Glycerine*
*1 tablespoon special orange
   flavoring (see page 210)*

1 1/2 cups brown rice flour
1 teaspoon baking soda
1 teaspoon ground cinnamon
1/4 teaspoon sea salt (optional)
*1/2 cup chopped or ground
   fresh walnuts (see note)*

Preheat oven to 375°F. Mix pumpkin, butter, glycerine, and orange flavoring in a large bowl. Add flour, baking soda, and seasonings; mix. Fold in nuts. Place teaspoonfuls on a nonstick cookie sheet. Bake 8–10 minutes, or until lightly browned. Let cookies stand for 5 minutes before removing them from cookie sheet. They will harden as they cool.

8 carbohydrates each

Note: If your digestive system is sensitive, try ground nuts rather than chopped, or omit altogether.

Scrumptious Rice Ball Cookies

YIELDS 2 DOZEN COOKIES

The texture and flavor of these plan-ahead cookies are marvelous!

1 cup brown rice flour
2 tablespoons Easy Clarified
  Butter (page 37)
1/4 cup 100% Pure Vegetable
  Glycerine

1 teaspoon special vanilla
  flavoring (see page 210)
2 large eggs, lightly beaten
1 cup ground fresh walnuts

Preheat oven to 375°F. Mix all ingredients in a medium bowl. Refrigerate several hours or overnight to allow flavors to blend. Roll dough into small balls; place on a nonstick cookie sheet. Bake 8–10 minutes. Let stand for 5 minutes before removing them from cookie sheet. Cookies will harden as they cool.

8 carbohydrates each

Note: These cookies freeze well.

Tarliki Cookies

YIELDS APPROXIMATELY 2½ DOZEN COOKIES

This delightful, delicate Middle-Eastern cookie recipe, courtesy of Ida W. Klinger, Albuquerque, New Mexico.

2 large eggs
1/4 cup Easy Clarified Butter
  (page 37)
2 tablespoons 100% Pure Vege-
  table Glycerine
1 teaspoon special vanilla
  flavoring (see page 210)

2 1/2 cups sifted brown rice
  flour, divided
1/2 cup arrowroot powder
1 teaspoon baking powder
1 egg white
1/4 cup sesame seeds

Preheat oven to 350°F. Place eggs, butter, glycerine, and flavoring in a large bowl; beat. Mix 2 cups flour, the arrowroot, and the baking powder in another bowl. Add mixture to eggs; blend. Cover; chill 1 hour. Add remaining ½ cup flour; mix. Roll on floured board; cut strips of dough, ¼ × 3 inches long; seal ends, forming a circle. Beat egg white in a small bowl; place sesame seeds in another bowl. Dip circles into egg white, then into seeds; place on a nonstick baking sheet. Bake 8–10 minutes.

17 carbohydrates each

Favorite Flan (Custard)

YIELDS 6 SERVINGS

This marvelous custard gets its delicious flavor from special maple flavoring.

2 cups unsweetened soy milk
  (see note)
2 tablespoons fresh lemon juice
1 cinnamon stick or 2 teaspoons
  ground cinnamon
8 egg yolks

¹/4 cup 100% Pure Vegetable
  Glycerine
2 teaspoons special maple
  flavoring (see page 210)
¹/2 teaspoon special vanilla
  flavoring

Preheat oven to 325°F. Heat milk, lemon juice, and cinnamon stick or ground cinnamon in a 2-quart nonstick saucepan, stirring frequently, until almost boiling (do not boil). Remove from heat; cool. Remove cinnamon stick. Beat egg yolks until creamy. Add cooled milk mixture, glycerine, and maple and vanilla flavorings to eggs; mix. Pour egg mixture into custard cups; set into a large baking dish with water. Bake 1 hour, or until firm. Refrigerate 1 hour before serving.

22 carbohydrates per serving

Note: If your digestive system is sensitive to soy, nut milk or egg whites may be used instead (see "Dairy Substitutes").

Royal Vanilla Custard

YIELDS 4 SERVINGS

Easy, delicious—and great "comfort food" for the tummy.

4 large eggs
1 cup unsweetened soy milk (see note)
1 tablespoon 100% Pure Vegetable Glycerin (page 37), melted

1 tablespoon special vanilla flavoring (see page 210)
Ground nutmeg

Preheat oven to 350°F. Place eggs in a food processor or beat with electric mixer. Add milk, glycerine and flavoring; mix well. Pout mixture into 4 custard cups; sprinkle tops with nutmeg. Set cups into a large baking dish with water. Bake for 30 to 33 minutes. Toothpick test. Cool; chill for 1 hour before serving.

17 carbohydrates per serving

Note: If you're sensitive to soy, nut milk or egg whites may be used instead (see "Dairy Substitutes).

Sunny Lemon Pudding

YIELDS 6 SERVINGS

You'll love this combination of tart and sweet flavors.

3 large egg yolks
3 tablespoons + 1 teaspoon arrowroot powder
1 cup water (purified, preferably), divided

2 teaspoons special lemon flavoring (see page 210)
3 tablespoons 100% Pure Vegetable Glycerine

Heat egg yolks and arrowroot in the top of a double boiler or nonstick saucepan. Gradually add 1/2 cup water; mix with a whisk over medium heat until thick. Add remaining 1/2 cup water and lemon flavoring, whisking until thick again. Remove from heat; cool. Add glycerine; stir. Spoon into 6 individual cups; chill 1 hour before serving.

4 carbohydrates per serving

Perfect Pecan Crust

YIELDS ONE 8-INCH PIECRUST OR 6 SERVINGS

This pecan crust is a delicious substitute for flour crust.

1/4 cup Easy Clarified Butter (page 37)   *1 cup ground fresh pecans*

Melt butter in a small skillet; remove from heat. Add pecans; stir. Spoon mixture into a greased, 8-inch pie dish, pressing against sides and bottom of dish to form crust. Fill and bake or chill according to filling instructions.

16 carbohydrates

Superb Oat Crust

YIELDS ONE 8-INCH PIECRUST OR 6 SERVINGS

This tasty substitute crust complements any pie filling

$1^1/2$ cups natural rolled oats
$1/2$ cup Easy Clarified Butter (page 37), melted
2 tablespoons 100% Pure Vegetable Glycerine

2 teaspoons ground cinnamon
$1/4$ teaspoon sea salt (optional)

Combine all ingredients in a medium-size mixing bowl; mix. Spoon mixture into an 8-inch pie dish, pressing against sides and bottom of dish to form crust. Fill and bake or chill according to filling instructions.

12 carbohydrates per serving

Lemon Meringue Pie

YIELDS 6 SERVINGS

No need to give up this family and company pleasing dessert!

3 large eggs
3 tablespoons + 1 teaspoon
*   arrowroot powder*
1 cup water (purified, preferably)
2 teaspoons Bickford's lemon
*   flavoring*

3 tablespoons 100% Pure Vege-
*   table Glycerine*
Perfect Pecan Crust (page 193)
Meringue Topping (page 197)

Separate eggs. Place yolks and arrowroot powder into the top of a double boiler; add water and flavoring. Using a whisk, mix over medium heat until thick. Remove from heat; cool. Add glycerine; stir. Pour into crust. Cover with Meringue Topping. Bake in 400° oven for 10 minutes or until delicately brown. Chill at least 2 hours before serving.

7 carbohydrates per serving

My Special Pumpkin Pie

YIELDS 6 SERVINGS

This pie recipe *proves* that you can be on the diet and still enjoy delicious desserts!

2 large eggs
2 cups canned unsweetened
*   pumpkin*
3 tablespoons 100% Pure Vege-
*   table Glycerine*
1¼ cups unsweetened soy milk
*   (see note)*

1 teaspoon each ground cinna-
*   mon and ginger*
¼ teaspoon ground cloves
½ teaspoon sea salt (optional)
Perfect Pecan Crust (page 193)
Special Cream Topping (page 197)

Preheat oven to 425°F. Beat eggs in a large bowl; stir in pumpkin, glycerine, milk, spices, and salt. Beat with electric mixer at high speed for 2 minutes; pour mixture into Perfect Pecan Crust. Bake 10 minutes. Reduce heat to 350°; bake 45 minutes more, or until firm. Cool; top with Special Cream Topping. Chill before serving.

25 carbohydrates per serving

Note: If you're sensitive to soy, nut milk or egg whites may be used instead (see "Dairy Substitutes").

Pecan Pie Royale

YIELDS 6 SERVINGS

Yes, it is even possible to have this special pecan pie on the diet. Delicious results!

3 eggs
¹/3 cup Easy Clarified Butter (page 37)
¹/2 cup 100% Pure Vegetable Glycerine
¹/4 teaspoon sea salt (optional)

1 teaspoon special vanilla flavoring (see page 210)
1¹/2 cups chopped fresh pecans (see note)
Superb Oat Crust (page 193)

Preheat oven to 375°F. Place eggs in a medium-sized mixing bowl; beat well. Add butter and glycerine, salt and flavoring; mix. Stir in pecans. Pour mixture into crust. Bake 25–30 minutes. Toothpick test. Cool slightly. Serve warm or chilled.

6 carbohydrates per serving

Note: If your digestive system is sensitive, try ground nuts, or omit altogether.

Almond and Butter Cream Icing

YIELDS TOPPING FOR 8-INCH CAKE

This is a perfect icing for Lemon Cake Supreme (page 184).

*½ cup + 2 tablespoons Easy
   Clarified Butter (page 37),
   melted
5 tablespoons 100% Pure Vegetable Glycerine*

*1 egg yolk
2 tablespoons fresh lemon juice
½ cup sliced or ground almonds
   (see note)*

Cream butter with glycerine. Beat in egg yolk and lemon juice; mix until thick. Fold almonds into icing or wait until cake is frosted and sprinkle over top.

16 carbohydrates

Note: Ground nuts are easier to digest than sliced.

Cinnamon-Nut Topping

YIELDS TOPPING FOR 1 DOZEN ROLLS

A delicious sugar-free topping for rolls.

*¼ cup Easy Clarified Butter
   (page 37)
½ cup ground fresh pecans or
   walnuts*

*1 tablespoon 100% Pure Vege-
   table Glycerine
1 teaspoon ground cinnamon, or
   more, to taste*

Melt butter in a small skillet. Add nuts, glycerine, and cinnamon; mix. Remove from heat; cool before spreading.

8 carbohydrates

Meringue Topping
YIELDS TOPPING FOR ONE 8-INCH OR 9-INCH PIE

This delightful topping uses a permitted sweetener and special flavoring with wonderful results!

2 large egg whites
1 tablespoon 100% Pure Vege-
table Glycerine

¹/₄ teaspoon special vanilla
flavoring (see page 210)

Preheat oven to 400°F. Beat whites until stiff. Fold in glycerine and vanilla. Spoon over pie filling. Bake 10 minutes, or until browned.

0 carbohydrates

Pancake Syrup Surprise
YIELDS APPROXIMATELY ¼ CUP

Glycerine and maple flavoring make this a delicious and easy-to-prepare syrup for pancakes and crepes.

¹/₄ cup 100% Pure Vegetable
Glycerine

1 teaspoon special maple
flavoring (see page 210)

Pour glycerine and flavoring into a small bowl; mix. Pour mixture into a small cream pitcher and serve.

0 carbohydrates

Pecan Custard Topping

YIELDS TOPPING FOR ONE 8-INCH CAKE

This topping is especially delicious spread over Best Poppy Seed Cake (page 183), a family favorite.

*½ cup unsweetened soy milk
(see note)
1 large egg yolk
1 tablespoon arrowroot powder
2 tablespoons 100% Pure Vegetable Glycerine*

*⅛ teaspoon sea salt (optional)
2 ounces chopped or ground
fresh pecans (see note)*

Place all ingredients, except nuts, in a double boiler or small nonstick saucepan. Heating to medium-high, mix ingredients with a whisk, keeping mixture smooth; then add pecans. Stir until thick enough to spread over cake. Cool before spreading.

4 carbohydrates

Note: If you're sensitive to soy, nut milk or egg whites may be used instead (see ''Dairy Substitutes''). If your digestive system is sensitive, use ground pecans instead of chopped.

Special Cream Topping
YIELDS TOPPING FOR AN 8-INCH PIE

Wonderful substitutions, such as raw cottage cheese, glycerine sweetener, and vanilla flavoring, make a delicious pie topping.

1 cup raw cottage cheese (see note)
1/4 cup plain low-fat yogurt
2 tablespoons 100% Pure Vegetable Glycerine

1 teaspoon special vanilla flavoring (see page 210)

Place all ingredients in a food processor or electric mixer; blend until smooth. Spoon over pie filling. Chill at least 30 minutes before serving.

11 carbohydrates

Note: If you have digestive problems, do not use raw cottage cheese. Drained fresh tofu, if tolerated, may be used instead.

Sweet Pecan Spread
YIELDS APPROXIMATELY ½ CUP

The fresh pecans and glycerine sweetener are a delicious combination. This easy-to-prepare spread may be used as a topping for rice cakes, rice crackers, or for Cinnamon and Nut Rolls (page 158).

1/4 pound fresh pecans

1 tablespoon 100% Pure Vegetable Glycerine

Finely chop nuts in a food processor or blender. Add glycerine; mix until smooth, but not too liquid. A delicious spread is ready!

8 carbohydrates

Why *Candida* Sufferers May Not Make a Full Recovery

1. Diet. *Candida* sufferers may not be on the *Candida* Control Diet consistently and/or for a long enough period of time.

2. Herbal Remedy or Medication. *Candida* sufferers may not be on the proper product, or a high enough dosage, consistently for a sufficient period of time.

3. Parasites. Many people who suffer from *Candida* also have parasites. Many times parasites may not show up in a routine stool culture because they live in the mucous of the intestines and colon. Two tests have been found to be useful: The Rectal Swab test, performed by a physician, and the Purged Stool test, which the patient does at home from a test kit supplied by the health care professional.

4. Thyroid Dysfunction. Many *Candida* sufferers have thyroid dysfunction. A full-panel thyroid test has been found to be useful for detection.

5. Allergies. There may be allergies to foods, molds, chemicals or other environmental factors. It has been found that it is beneficial to alternate foods—to not have the same food for several days to keep an allergy from building up.

6. *Candida albicans* Allergy. Some *Candida* sufferers may be allergic to the *Candida* yeast itself. There is a test for this, and an antigen is available.

7. Secretory IGA (protective saliva). Some sufferers may not produce enough secretory IGA. Testing is available.

8. Mercury in Silver Amalgams. There is evidence to show that there is enough mecury in silver amalgams (tooth fillings)—50%—to cause problems for many *Candida* sufferers. If the silver amalgams are to be changed, they should be removed by a dentist who is familiar with removing mercury. During removal, a dam in the mouth may insure that the patient doesn't ingest the mercury. It has been found that removal should be done very carefully and gradually, not less than one month between procedures. In addition, the new material should be tested for patient sensitivity.

9. Stress. If the same excessive or continued emotional stress is present that was there at the onset of illness, the problem must be addressed for a full recovery. Many times work situations or relationships have to be changed. If the patient cannot alleviate the stress, counseling may help.

10. Attitude. It is extremely important to get rid of any negative attitudes and instead to try to develop a positive one in order to make a good recovery. It also is necessary to try to surround oneself with very positive, supportive friends, and even new ones if necessary. Many new friends and good support can be found at a *Candida* support group. The Candida Research and Information Foundation has a list of *Candida* support groups which may be in your area. To obtain the Foundation's address, see Appendix C.

It takes a great deal of determination, hard work and much perseverance to conquer *Candida*, but it is worth it!

Appendix A
Nutritional Supplements
for the *Candida* Condition

The following supplements have been found to be beneficial for *Candida* conditions and are available over the counter in most health and natural food stores. A note of caution: *Avoid supplements with a* **yeast base.**

Anti-fungal Agents are beneficial to the patient in reducing the toxins produced by *Candida*.

Butyric acid (available in capsules) has been shown to heal mucous membranes that have been damaged by *Candida*.

Caprylic acid (available in capsules, liquid, or tablets), a short-chain fatty acid that has been found to be anti-fungal for *Candida* and other fungi. It is found in mother's milk, but the commercial form is derived from coconut.

Cayenne pepper is excellent for digestion and circulation; this herb has been reported to be anti-fungal and anti-parasitic.

Garlic is beneficial in any form for killing yeast.

La Pacho is a tea made from the inner bark of trees grown in South American rain forests that do not grow fungi. This tea has been beneficial for numerous *Candida* patients both when used internally and when used topically for skin fungal infections.

Lauric acid (available in capsules) is derived from coconut oil. This acid alters the cell wall of *Candida*, allowing the body to destroy the organism.

Mycocidin (available in capsules) is derived from castor oil. This product has proven extremely effective as an anti-fungal agent used against *Candida* symptomology.

Propionic acid (available in capsules or tablets), a short-chain fatty acid derived by bacterial fermentation, works as an anti-fungal agent on all forms of *Candida*.

Tanalbit (available in capsules) is a combination of zinc and tannate derived from plant source natural bioflavonoids—which are both fat and lipid soluble. Tanalbit destroys the cell wall of *Candida*; tannate heals mucous membranes and aids in removal of immunosuppressant mercury from tissues.

Flora-Replacing Bacteria/Immunity Builders The flora-replacing bacteria aid in digestion, in supporting the immune system and other bodily functions of *Candida* patients. Immunity builders are products that have been found to stimulate the immune systems of *Candida* patients.

Acidophilus (available in capsules, liquid or powder) *Bifidus* (available in powder) *Streptococcus fecium* (available in capsules or powder) — Bacteria shown by research to inhibit dissemination of *Candida* and other fungi through the intestinal wall; also inhibits *Candida* attachment to mucosa.

Aloe vera (available in liquid) aids in healing mucous membranes and soothing stomach or intestinal burning of *Candida* and other patients with parasitic problems. Notes of caution: *Use pure aloe vera only. This product can cause diarrhea.*

Biotin (available capsules or tablets) is a B vitamin normally produced by the bowel flora, keeps *Candida* in its simpler form, which is easier to eliminate. A biotin deficiency allows for *Candida* or yeast overgrowth.

Germanium sesquioxide (available capsules, powder or tablets) is one of the natural elements found to oxygenate the human system; also acts as an immune stimulant. This product has been beneficial in *Candida* treatment.

Iron (available in tablets) is essential to health. If a person has *Candida* and is also iron deficient, the deficiency must be corrected before the *Candida* can be eliminated. A note of caution: *Only to be used to replace diagnosed deficiencies. Avoid taking in excess!*

Magnesium (available in capsules or tablets) is another essential mineral. Many *Candida* patients have been found to be magnesium deficient. Magnesium controls many of the biochemical functions in the body and is essential for *Candida* recovery.

Oelic and linolenic acids (available capsules or liquid) are derived from essential fats, such as evening primrose oil, olive oil, and fish oils that are necessary for many bodily functions.

Zinc (available tablets) is an important cofactor for uptake of all nutrients, as well as immunostimulating for *Candida* patients.

Short- to Medium-Chain Fatty Acids have specific antifungal properties for the condition created by *Candida*.

Butyric acid (in capsules) heals *Candida*-damaged mucous membranes.

Caprylic acid (in capsules, liquid, or tablets) is anti-fungal for *Candida* and other fungi.

Mycocidin (in capsules) is an anti-fungal agent for *Candida* symptomology.

Propionic acid (in capsules or tablets) is an anti-fungal agent on all forms of *Candida*.

Long-Chain Fatty Acids are important in general homeostasis, or balance of the systems of the body, and in the integrity of the immune system of the *Candida* patient.

Cod liver oil (available in capsules or liquid) heals damaged mucous membranes and restores integrity in the gastrointestinal system of the *Candida* patient.

EPA (available in capsules) is a fish oil that provides important Omega-3 fatty acids in *Candida* treatment.

Evening primrose oil (available in capsules or liquid) provides substantial amounts of Omega-6 fatty acid—gamma linolenic acid—which is often deficient in *Candida* patients.

Nutritional linseed oil (available in capsules or liquid) is derived from flax seed and provides essential fatty acids necessary for improving bodily functions of *Candida* patients.

Olive oil (available as liquid) is a mono oil that provides essential fatty acids and doesn't change its molecular structure under moderate heat—which is beneficial for *Candida* conditions.

Rapeseed oil (available in liquid) is a mono oil that does not change its molecular structure when heated and is therefore beneficial for *Candida* cooking.

Digestive Aids Research shows that *Candida* patients may have poor digestion. These digestive aids have been found to be beneficial:

Hydrochloric acid (available in capsules or tablets)
Pancreatic enzymes (available in capsules or tablets)   Aid in digestion where impaired by *Candida* infection.
Whole food enzymes (available in capsules)

A note of caution: *Hydrochloric acid, in liquid form, is not recommended because of possible damage to teeth enamel.*

Anti-oxidants block the effects of toxins caused by *Candida*. These toxins are highly unstable and are capable of causing cellular damage.

Beta carotene (available in capsules or tablets) is a natural form of vitamin A which the body converts to usable A. Many *Candida* patients have been found to be deficient in usable A. Beta carotene has also been found to be protective at the cellular level.

Dimethylglycine (DMG) or vitamin B_{15} (available in tablets that dissolve under the tongue) is a potent anti-oxidant that helps liver detoxify chemicals.

Selenium (available in capsules, liquid, or tablets) is a major anti-oxidant; an essential mineral that protects against *Candida* toxins.

Vitamin A (available in capsules or tablets) is a fat-soluble vitamin, best taken with fresh vegetables, which will provide the enzymes necessary for its uptake by the body; aids in healing *Candida* damage to the membranes.

Vitamin C (available in capsules, liquid, or tablets) enhances the immune system and protects against damage by toxic products of *Candida*.

Vitamin E (available in capsules or liquid) heals mucous membranes; protects against toxins of *Candida*.

Antifungal Douche Formulas—These formulas reduce the *Candida* population: Bee Kind, Yeast Gard, and Orithrush are some of the products that are used vaginally for yeast infections. Sero-Aseptic is used both orally, as a gargle, and vaginally for yeast infections.

As you can see, there are many beneficial nutritional supplements for the *Candida* condition. However, since each individual and each condition are different, it is essential for a health care professional to determine your dosage and to monitor all aspects of your treatment program.

Appendix B
Products and Sources

The products in this section should be ordered through your health or natural food store or coop. Manufacturers and distributors will not sell to individuals. Note: If a particular brand listed here is not obtainable, choose another that has a similar description.

Agar-Agar (seaweed gelatin, substitute for animal gelatin, without antibiotics or steroids)

SOURCES: Eden Foods, Inc.
701 Tecumseh Road
Clinton, MI 49236
(800) 248-0301

Arrowroot Powder (cornstarch substitute for corn sensitivity)

SOURCES: Nature's Best
P.O. Box 2248
Brea, CA 92822
(800) 765-3141

Bread and Bakery Goods

Brown rice bread (100% wheat and yeast-free)
Kamut bread (100% wheat and yeast-free)
Millet bread (100% wheat and yeast-free)
Rye bread (100% wheat and yeast-free)
Sourdough bread (100% yeast-free)
Spelt bread, bagels and pizza crust (all 100% wheat and yeast-free)

SOURCE: French Meadow Bakery
2610 Lyndale Avenue South
Minneapolis, MN 55408
(612) 870-4740

Brown Rice (organic, short grain, preferably)

SOURCE: Arrowhead Mills, Inc.
          P.O. Box 2059
          Hereford, TX 79045
          (800) 749-0730

Brown Rice Chips/Crackers (wheatless, contain no tamari or fruit sweeteners)

Brown Rice Chips

SOURCES: Amsnack, Inc.
         7770 Longe Street
         Stockton, CA 95206
         (209) 982-5545

Brown Rice Wafers

Sources: Westbrae Natural Foods
          P.O. Box 48006
          Gardena, CA 90248
          (800) 776-1276

Cereals (without fruit, honey, malt, molasses, sugar, wheat, or yeast)

Puffed Rice
Rice and Shine
Oat Bran

SOURCES: Arrowhead Mills, Inc.
         P.O. Box 2059
         Hereford, TX 79045
         (806) 749-0730

Mother's Oat Bran
Quaker Puffed Rice

SOURCE: The Quaker Oats Company
          P.O. Box 049003
          Chicago, IL 60604-9003
          (312) 222-7111

Cheese (unsweetened, no mold, citric acid or other chemicals)

Caution: Only use if tolerated.

Stueve's Natural Raw Cottage Cheese

SOURCES: Alta Dena Dairies
P.O. Box 388
City of Industry, CA 91747
(800) 535-1369

Chicken Broth (unsweetened, no preservatives or chemicals)

Hain 100% Naturals Chicken Broth

SOURCE: The Hain Food Group
Natural Food Division
225 Carob Street
Compton, CA 90220
(800) 776-1276

Cranberry Concentrate (natural, unsweetened, no preservatives)

Just Cranberry by Knudsen

SOURCES: Knudsen & Sons, Inc.
P.O. Box 369
Chico, CA 95927
(530) 899-5010

Flavorings (no alcohol, sugar, or salt)

The Spicery Shoppe Non-Alcoholic Flavorings

SOURCE: The Spicery Shoppe
1525 Brook Drive
Downers Grove, IL 60515
1-800-323-1301

Flours (wheatless, no gluten)

Amaranth, buckwheat, corn, garbanzo bean, millet, potato, rice and soy

SOURCE: Arrowhead Mills, Inc.
     P.O. Box 2059
     Hereford, TX 79045
     (800) 749-0730

Garbanzo Beans (chickpeas), organically grown

SOURCE: Arrowhead Mills
     P.O. Box 2059
     Hereford, TX 79045
     (806) 749-0730

Olive Oil (100% pure, cold-pressed or expeller-pressed)

SOURCE: The Hain Food Group
     Natural Food Division
     225 Carob Street
     Compton, CA 90220
     (800) 776-1276

Pasta

Bifun (100% wheat-free Chinese noodles)

SOURCE: Eden Foods, Inc.
        701 Tecumseh Road
        Clinton, MI 49236
        (800) 248-0301

Corn Pasta (angel hair, elbows, garden twist, shells and spaghetti)

Caution: Do not eat above pasta if sensitive to corn.

SOURCE: Westbrae Natural Foods
        P. O. Box 48006
        Gardena, CA 90248
        (800) 776-1276

Harasume (Japanese rice noodles)

Kuzu-Kiri (Japanese clear noodles)

Soba (100% pure buckwheat Japanese noodles)

SOURCE: Eden Foods, Inc.
        701 Tecumseh Road
        Clinton, MI 49236
        (800) 248-0301

Quinoa (pronouced KEEN-WA, is mother grain, contains more protein than any other grain, and is easy to digest)

SOURCES: Eden Foods, Inc.
        701 Tecumseh Road
        Clinton, MI 49236
        (800) 248-0301

        Nature's Best
        P.O. Box 2248
        Brea, CA 92822
        (800) 765-3141

Rice Cakes

Lundberg Rice Cakes (brown rice cakes)

SOURCES: Lundberg Family Farms
P.O. Box 369
Richvale, CA 95974
(530) 882-4551

Mochi (Japanese rice cake)

SOURCE: Grainaissance, Inc.
1580 62nd Street
Emeryville, CA 94608
(800) 472-4697

Safflower Oil (100% pure, cold-pressed or expeller-pressed)

SOURCE: The Hain Food Group
Natural Food Division
225 Carob Street
Compton, CA 90220
(800) 776-1276

Sea Salt (free of chemicals and sweeteners)

La Baleine Sea Salt

SOURCES: Gourmet France
9355 Remick Avenue
Arleta, CA 91331
(818) 768-4300

Sesame Tahini (certified organic, mechanically hulled sesame seeds)

SOURCE: Maranatha Natural Foods, Inc.
P.O. Box 1046
Ashland, OR 97520
(541) 488-2747

Soy Milk

Pure Soyquick

SOURCES: Ener-G Foods, Inc.
P.O. Box 84487
Seattle, WA 98124-5787
(800) 331-5222

West Soy
SOURCES: Nature's Best
P.O. Box 2248
Brea, CA 92822
(800) 765-3141

Taheebo Tea (also known as Pau D'Arco, La pacho, Ipe Roxo, Tabeuia, Tecoma, Bow Stick).

This tea is from the bark of trees grown in the rain forests of South America, is free of fungus, and is a natural antifungal for Candida and CRC treatment.

SOURCES: Alta Health Products
1979 East Locust Street
Pasadena, CA 91107
(800) 423-4155

Tomatoes

Pomi Chopped Tomatoes and Strained Tomatoes (no salt added, no artificial flavoring, water or preservatives. Not from concentrate; packaged from fresh tomatoes)

SOURCE: Parmalat U.S.A. Corp.
400 Frank W. Burr Blvd.
Teaneck, NJ 07666
(800) 831-7664

Note: If this brand or similar description is not obtainable, it is best to use fresh tomatoes, scrubbing them first before cutting or pureeing for sauces.

Vegetable Glycerine 100% Pure, (See page 34)

Sources: Starwest Botanicals
11253 Trade Center Drive
Rancho Cordova, CA 95742
(800) 800-4372

Vegetables (frozen, unsweetened, and contain no preservatives, chemicals, or pesticides. Includes corn*, green beans, mixed vegetables, peas, spinach.)

Sources: Sno Pac Foods, Inc.
521 West Enterprise
Caledonia, MN 55921
(800) 533-2215

*Many people are sensitive to corn. *Eat with caution.*

Appendix C
Candida & Dysbiosis
Information Foundation
(Formerly The Candida Research
and Information Foundation)

The Foundation is a world-wide private, non-profit organization. It works with physicians and patients from around the world; its goal is to let others know that there is hope and help for those suffering from chronic health problems. The Foundation is committed to providing current and accurate information on the subject of yeast and its relationship to human health, and to aid suffers in obtaining the necessary help to regain and maintain good health. The Foundation provides lists of doctors who treat *Candida,* as well as informative newsletters about progress and reading lists on the treatment of Candidiasis. Emotional help is given individually or through support groups. Counseling is also available for dealing with *Candida*-related problems. Meetings are also organized with speakers on Candida-related subjects.

The long-term goal of the Foundation is to facilitate and financially support research aiding in the diagnosis of *Candida,* to identify those biochemical factors that set the stage for *Candida* infection and ultimately to eradicate Candidiasis as a problem in human health.

For further information, please write to:

C.D.I.F.
P. O. Box JF
College Station, TX 77841-5146
Telephone: (409) 694-8687

References

Bosco, Dominick and Rosenbaum, Michael E., *Super Supplements*. Signet, 1989.

Chaitow, Leon, *Candida Albicans: Could Yeast be Your Problem?* Thorsons Publishing Group, 1985.

Connoloy, Pat and Associates of the Price Pottenger Nutrition Foundation, *The Candida Albicans Yeast-Free Cookbook*. Keats Publishing, Inc., 1985.

Crook, William G., M.D., *The Yeast Connection*. Jackson, Tennessee: Professional Books, 1985.

Higa, Barbara W. And Remington, Dennis W., *Back to Health: A Comprehensive Medical and Nutritional Yeast-Control Program*. Vitality House International, Inc., 1986

Lorenzani, Shirley S., Ph.D., *Candida: A Twentieth-Century Disease*. New Canaan, Connecticut: Keats Publishing, Inc., 1986.

Rosenbaum, Michael, M.D. and Susser, Murray, M.D., *Solving the Puzzle of Chronic Fatigue Syndrome*. Tacoma, Washington: Life Science Press, 1992.

Trowbridge, John Parks and Walker, Morton, *The Yeast Syndrome*. Bantam Books, 1986.

Truss, C. Orian, M.D., *The Missing Diagnosis*, Birmingham, Alabama: C.O. Truss, 1983.

United States Department of Agriculture, *Nutritive Value of American Foods in Common Units*. Agriculture Handbook #456, 1975.

Index